INTRODUCTION TO
HEALTH INFORMATION
PRIVACY AND SECURITY

Laurie A. Rinehart-Thompson
JD, RHIA, CHP, FAHIMA

ISBN: 978-1-58426-353-1
AHIMA Product No.: AB109912

AHIMA Staff:
Jessica Block, MA, Assistant Editor
Jason O. Malley, Director, Creative Content Development
Ashley R. Sullivan, Production Development Editor
Angela Rose, MHA, RHIA, CHPS, Reviewer
Diana Warner, MS, RHIA, CHPS, FAHIMA, Reviewer

For more information, including updates, about AHIMA Press publications, visit http://www.ahima.org/publications/updates.aspx.

American Health Information Management Association
233 North Michigan Avenue, 21st Floor
Chicago, Illinois 60601-5809
ahima.org

Contents

Online Resource: Student Workbook

Detailed Contents

About the Author

Laurie A. Rinehart-Thompson, JD, RHIA, CHP, FAHIMA, is an associate professor of clinical health and rehabilitation sciences in the Health Information Management and Systems program at The Ohio State University, Columbus, OH. She earned her Bachelor of Science degree in medical record administration and her Juris Doctor degree, both from The Ohio State University. In addition to education, her professional experiences span the behavioral health, home health, and acute care arenas. She has served as an expert witness in civil litigation, testifying as to the privacy and confidentiality of health information. She has served on the AHIMA CHP Exam Construction, Advocacy, and Policy, and Education Strategy Committees, and the AHIMA Privacy and Security Practice Council. She is currently a member of the AHIMA Professional Ethics Committee and the Research and Periodicals Workgroup of the Council on Excellence in Education. She has served twice on the Executive Board of Directors of the Ohio Health Information Management Association and is currently a project leader for its legislative strategy. She is a recipient of the AHIMA Triumph Award and the Ohio Health Information Management Association Distinguished Member Award. A frequent speaker on the HIPAA Privacy Rule, she is coeditor and coauthor of AHIMA's *Fundamentals of Law for Health Informatics and Information Management* Second Edition; and a contributing author to *Ethical Challenges in the Management of Health Information* Second Edition, copublished by AHIMA and Jones and Bartlett, AHIMA's *Health Information Management Technology: An Applied Approach* Fourth Edition, AHIMA's *Documentation for Medical Practices*, and the *Journal of AHIMA*. Her work has also been published in AHIMA's *Perspectives in Health Information Management*.

Preface

With the passage of the Health Insurance Portability and Accountability Act (HIPAA) in 1996 and the subsequent effective dates of the Privacy and Security Rules in 2003 and 2005, tremendous resources have been spent to both prepare for and ensure ongoing compliance with health information privacy and security regulations. As a result, much attention has been focused on the resulting outlay of both time and money. Therefore, it is important to look deeper at the objectives of these laws and their basic intent: to protect patient information and grant individuals rights pertaining to their protected health information. At a minimum, by studying this book the reader will learn the basic principles of the HIPAA Privacy and Security Rules. The reader will also appreciate the fact that health information tells the stories of people's lives. This is why health information warrants such necessary protections and why individual rights are so vital. This book is designed to introduce the HIPAA Privacy Rule and HIPAA Security Rule to the reader who has had little or no exposure to either or who simply wishes to refresh his understanding of the basics. It provides a reference for students enrolled in courses or programs of study that require a solid understanding of the Privacy and Security Rules. This can include students in any health-related academic program. The book also serves as an educational reference for health information technology certificate programs; Regional Extension Centers (RECs); consultants and other healthcare professionals; third-party payers; academic libraries; and workforce members in covered entities, business associate or subcontractor settings where little or no formal training has been provided about the principles of patient information privacy and security.

The text is presented in six chapters, beginning with an overview of health information regulation, followed by the presentation of key information related to the HIPAA Privacy Rule and the Security Rule, and closing with a discussion of key changes to the rules as created by the 2009 Health Information Technology for Economic and Clinical Health (HITECH) Act.

Chapter 1 discusses the many ways, both internal and external to an organization, that health information is regulated. In this chapter, the reader is introduced to forces that controlled the use and disclosure of patient information prior to HIPAA, and which continue to have an impact today. This chapter also discusses the concept of meaningful use, which plays a significant role in the certification and adoption of electronic health records (EHRs).

Chapter 2 introduces the reader to the scope of the HIPAA Privacy and Security Rules. It first identifies the broader context of the HIPAA law in which these rules exist, and then proceeds to describe terms of art specific to HIPAA that will guide the reader toward a greater understanding of the rules and the scope of who is covered (that is, who is legally obligated to adhere to them) and what is covered (that is, what information is protected).

Chapter 3 provides an overview of the HIPAA Privacy Rule by explaining key documents, addressing authorization requirements (and the many exceptions), and discussing preemption and the important rights to which individuals are entitled. The chapter concludes by explaining the Privacy Rule's provisions relating to marketing and fundraising activities, research, and administrative requirements.

Chapter 4 explains the structure of the HIPAA Security Rule, detailing its organization according to the physical, technical, and administrative safeguard standards as well as describing requirements for policies and procedures and documentation. Examples of implementation and specific items for consideration are provided for selected requirements.

Chapter 5 discusses the concept of business risks as they relate to health information. In a two-part process, the chapter will discuss risk analysis as the process of risk and asset identification followed by a discussion of contingency plans development to respond to risks that become reality. Both risk analysis and contingency planning are viewed through the lens of the HIPAA Security Rule, which requires that they be put into place.

Chapter 6 details the first major revision to the HIPAA Privacy and Security Rules since their creation: the Health Information Technology for Economic and Clinical Health (HITECH) Act, which became law as part of the American Recovery and Reinvestment Act (ARRA) of 2009. Because HITECH introduced large-scale changes through the introduction of administrative rules, this chapter first walks the reader through the federal rulemaking process. It describes various types of administrative rules and discusses federally required publication and review mechanisms. The reader will be introduced to HITECH's changes as they relate to the concepts introduced in chapters 2 and 3. They include business associates and subcontractors; breach notification; individual rights; the minimum necessary requirement; personal health record vendors; marketing; fundraising; sale of protected health information; increased enforcement and penalties for noncompliance; protected health information of decedents; research authorization requirements; student immunization requirements; and changes to the notice of privacy practices.

Each chapter contains Check Your Understanding questions and concludes with a Real-World Case that is derived from a news story or illustrates an issue relevant to the topics presented in the chapter. The reader will notice helpful resources in the text such as sample forms, figures that break concepts into manageable portions, and references to further the reader's understanding about specific topics. A complete glossary is also present at the end of the book. It supplements the key terms introduced in boldface type in each chapter to indicate the first substantial reference to them.

It is my sincere hope that, by delving into a study of HIPAA privacy and security, the reader develops an appreciation for the purpose of HIPAA as well as the committed efforts of the many healthcare professionals who work to uphold its intent each and every day.

Acknowledgments

The publisher thanks Deborah J. Perkins, RHIA, CPHQ, FACHE, FAHIMA, for her review and feedback on this book.

I dedicate this book to my husband, Tim; my sons, Noah and Joel; and my parents, Joseph and Betty Rinehart, for all their love and support. I thank Melanie Brodnik for her invaluable mentorship, and her tireless dedication to the health information management profession and the ideals of professionalism.

Laurie A. Rinehart-Thompson

Foreword

The issuance of privacy and security regulations under HIPAA has focused national attention more squarely on patients' rights to the confidential treatment of their health information. A great deal of study and effort has been expended over the past decade in bringing healthcare providers' and business associate practices into compliance with HIPAA's requirements. But no understanding of privacy and security can be complete without recognizing that privacy and security concerns existed prior to HIPAA, and continue to exist years after the healthcare industry began its work to comply with HIPAA's implementing regulations. As a professional beginning your study of privacy and security, you have taken a good first step by selecting this book, which offers a wonderful introduction to key aspects of the privacy and security landscape. I hope that once you have completed the book, you will be interested in continuing your study by exploring the nuances and challenges that continue to emerge as regulations change, new technologies and uses of health information emerge, and as we collectively discover (sometimes the hard way) what does and does not work in our methods of protecting health information.

These are not easy issues. The safe and appropriate use and disclosure of health information require not only an understanding of what is required, but also what is "right." State laws and regulations, ethical codes, accreditation standards, and even a strong focus on serving the patient all enter into making good decisions in handling health information. Reading this book is a positive move towards understanding what is required, and it should spark your interest in knowing more.

One of the most troubling practices I see in privacy and security compliance programs is the tendency for some working in the healthcare industry to rely exclusively on others' interpretations and opinions on the acceptability of certain information-handling practices, as a substitute for understanding the principles of privacy and security themselves. Because the acceptability of any practice really turns upon the specific facts involved, that kind of "hands-off" approach to privacy and security compliance results in bad decisions that hurt patients and put covered entities at risk. The fact that you have chosen this topic of study indicates that you may be part of the solution to that problem. So welcome to your study of privacy and security! We need you.

Jill Callahan Dennis, JD, RHIA
Past-President, AHIMA

CHAPTER 1

How Health Information Is Regulated

Learning Objectives

- Identify federal laws that regulate health information and distinguish the scope of their reach

- Describe preemption and explain situations when it does and does not apply

- Describe accreditation and certification, and identify and compare healthcare accreditation organizations

- Compare the electronic health record certification programs established by the Office of the National Coordinator for Health Information Technology

- Define meaningful use and explain how the Office of the National Coordinator for Health Information Technology's electronic health record certification programs promote meaningful use

- Describe the roles that professional ethical standards and organizational policies play in regulating the use and disclosure of health information

KEY TERMS

Accreditation

Accreditation Association for Ambulatory Health Care (AAAHC)

Administrative rule

American Health Information Management Association (AHIMA) Code of Ethics

American National Standards Institute (ANSI)

American Osteopathic Association (AOA)

American Recovery and Reinvestment Act (ARRA) of 2009

Centers for Medicare and Medicaid Services (CMS)

Certification

Certification Commission for Health Information Technology (CCHIT)

Child Abuse Prevention and Treatment Act (CAPTA) of 1996

Commission on Accreditation of Rehabilitation Facilities (CARF)

Comprehensive Alcohol Abuse and Alcoholism Prevention, Treatment, and Rehabilitation Act of 1970

Conditions of Participation (CoP)

Drug Abuse Prevention, Treatment, and Rehabilitation Act of 1972

Electronic Healthcare Network Accreditation Commission (EHNAC)

Freedom of Information Act (FOIA) of 1967

Health Information Technology for Economic and Clinical Health (HITECH) Act

Health Insurance Portability and Accountability Act (HIPAA) of 1996

Healthcare Effectiveness and Data Information Set (HEDIS)

Healthcare Facilities Accreditation Program (HFAP)

HIPAA Privacy Rule

HIPAA Security Rule

Joint Commission

Meaningful use

National Center for Health Statistics (NCHS)

National Committee for Quality Assurance (NCQA)

National Institute of Standards and Technology (NIST)

National Voluntary Laboratory Accreditation Program (NVLAP)

Office of the National Coordinator for Health Information Technology (ONC)

Office of the National Coordinator for Health Information Technology-Approved Accreditor (ONC-AA)

Office of the National Coordinator for Health Information Technology-Authorized Certification Body (ONC-ACB)

Office of the National Coordinator for Health Information Technology-Authorized Testing and Certification Body (ONC-ATCB)

Preemption

Privacy Act of 1974

Statute

United States Department of Health and Human Services (HHS)

INTRODUCTION

There are many ways that health information is regulated. The most familiar to many is the **Health Insurance Portability and Accountability Act of 1996 (HIPAA)**, a federal law enacted, in part, to provide federal protections for personal health information. However, prior to its passage and implementation, other federal and state laws existed that governed the use and disclosure of health information in a variety of ways. As will be discussed later in the text, already-existing laws must be evaluated to determine if they are consistent with HIPAA. If not, a legal determination must to be made about which law will be followed. Accreditation bodies, professional codes of ethics, and organizational policies also address the appropriate handling of health information. This chapter discusses the many ways that health information is regulated and how these regulations affect the handling of information. A detailed discussion of HIPAA is reserved for the remaining chapters of this book.

Section 1: Federal Laws

Today, when healthcare professionals think of health information regulation, they generally think of HIPAA. However, there are several federal laws that existed long before HIPAA that still exist today. They do not affect health information as broadly as HIPAA does. This section will discuss pre-HIPAA federal laws and will also introduce HIPAA and changes under the **Health Information Technology for Economic and Clinical Health Act (HITECH)**, which was enacted to promote the use of health information technology and to strengthen standards for the privacy and security of health information. HITECH is covered in greater detail in chapters 2 and 6.

Freedom of Information Act of 1967

The **Freedom of Information Act (FOIA) of 1967**, states that federal agency records should be disclosed to and accessed by the public (5 USC § 552). By openly sharing its records, the federal government is accountable to its citizens and, ultimately, its taxpayers. It is important for the public to be able to inspect the documents, and therefore the work, of the federal government. However, because some information is particularly sensitive and private there are exceptions to the general rule of access and disclosure. One exception is health records, if the reasons for disclosure do not outweigh the exception. This exception serves to preserve individuals' privacy. The law applies to healthcare providers owned and operated by the federal government. One example is the Department of Veterans Affairs. FOIA does not apply to healthcare organizations that are not owned and operated by the federal government (Brodnik et al. 2012).

Privacy Act of 1974

The **Privacy Act of 1974** "requires federal agencies holding personally identifiable records to safeguard that information and provide individuals with certain privacy rights," such as the right to access and request amendments to their records (Brodnik et al. 2012, 218). Although the purpose of this law is privacy and nondisclosure (as compared to FOIA, which promotes disclosure), it also applies to health information in a limited way because it only pertains to information collected by the federal government (for example, Department of Veterans Affairs facilities), and it does not specifically apply to health information.

Federal Drug and Alcohol Laws

The federal **Drug Abuse Prevention, Treatment, and Rehabilitation Act of 1972** and the **Comprehensive Alcohol Abuse and Alcoholism Prevention, Treatment, and Rehabilitation Act of 1970** specifically protect information relating to drug or other substance abuse. They protect information related to diagnosis, treatment of conditions, and referral for treatment (Brodnik et al. 2012). These laws apply more specifically to health information than the Privacy Act does because they apply to all federally assisted alcohol and drug abuse treatment programs, which includes more than just federal providers. However, they are limited because they only apply to a certain group of patients rather than to health information generally.

Medicare Conditions of Participation

In order to receive reimbursement from Medicare and Medicaid, providers must follow requirements called the **Conditions of Participation (CoP)**. The CoP require that the confidentiality of patient information be ensured. However, as with the previous federal laws discussed, the CoP are also limited. They regulate only providers who receive reimbursement from the Medicare and Medicaid programs. While this includes a large number of providers, the CoP do not apply to nonproviders who possess confidential patient information. The CoP also does not apply to patients insured by other payers or those not covered by insurance at all (Brodnik et al. 2012).

HIPAA and HITECH

The limited federal laws discussed previously protect only certain types of health information, such as drug and alcohol abuse records, or information held by certain entities, such as agencies of the federal government. Because they were not tailored to protect all types of patient information, they provide insufficient patient privacy protections. Further, state laws that protect patient information are inconsistent. As a result, prior to HIPAA, many types of health information were not protected by any law. After several attempts to create a uniform federal law that protected health information, Congress enacted HIPAA, which is a **statute**. A statute is a law that a legislative body, such as Congress, passes. The **HIPAA Privacy Rule**, an administrative law created by the **United States Department of Health and Human Services (HHS)**, which stems from the HIPAA statute passed by Congress, took effect in April 2003. An **administrative rule**, which is administrative law, provides greater detail than the statute from which it is created. An administrative rule enables a statute to be implemented or carried out. The HIPAA Privacy Rule protects all types of health information equally and affects more entities than other laws do (Brodnik et al. 2012). It is limited as well, because it only applies to healthcare providers that conduct defined electronic transactions. The Privacy Rule counterpart, the **HIPAA Security Rule**, regulates electronic health information and took effect in April 2005. HIPAA has had a remarkable effect on how people view the privacy and security of patient information. This text will refer to the HIPAA statute, Privacy Rule, and Security Rule only as HIPAA unless further delineation is necessary.

On February 17, 2009, President Obama signed the **American Recovery and Reinvestment Act (ARRA)**, a statute. In addition to health information technology funding and economic stimulus funding, it made changes to the HIPAA Privacy and Security Rules. These changes are located in HITECH, a statute within ARRA. The compliance date for HITECH provisions affecting HIPAA was February 17, 2010, which was one year after the law was signed, but varying timelines have created multiple compliance deadlines (Brodnik et al. 2012).

Section 2: State Laws

Recognizing the Role of State Law

Except for limited federal laws, state laws protected private patient information and governed access, use, and disclosure prior to HIPAA. State laws varied considerably, creating a patchwork effect. While many states passed laws to protect highly sensitive health information such as behavioral health and HIV or AIDS, not all states possessed laws that protected health information generally. When the HIPAA Privacy Rule took effect, a minimum amount of protection (that is, a floor) was achieved uniformly across all the states through a consistent set of requirements that affected many entities holding health information.

Even with HIPAA, healthcare professionals must be aware of state laws that affect access, use, and disclosure of health information. Subject to preemption, which is discussed in the following section, state laws are still in effect and laws provide important special protections to many sensitive information above and beyond what HIPAA provides (Brodnik et al. 2012).

Understanding Preemption

The legal doctrine of **preemption** applies to HIPAA. Although there is a legal obligation to comply with both state and federal privacy laws, sometimes an organization or individual cannot comply with both. To address this conflict, the preemption doctrine requires compliance with federal law when federal and state laws conflict. In other words, federal law preempts or supersedes state law that is contrary. A state law is contrary when it would be impossible to follow both a federal and a state law or when the state law is an obstacle to accomplishing the purpose of the federal law—in this case, HIPAA (45 CFR Part 160 Subpart B).

What if state law goes above and beyond so that it provides greater patient privacy protection than HIPAA does? Because HIPAA only provides a minimum (floor) of privacy protections and the goal is to provide as much protection as possible, HIPAA would not preempt the stricter (more stringent) state law in that case. More stringent means that the state law either provides individuals with greater privacy protections or it gives individuals greater rights regarding their own protected health information (Brodnik et al. 2012).

There are some situations where state law will not be preempted by HIPAA, even if the state law is not more stringent. Figure 1.1 illustrates these situations.

FIGURE 1.1.	Situations where state law is not preempted by HIPAA

The HIPAA Privacy Rule will not preempt state law if state law fulfills one or more of the following purposes:

1. Is determined by the Secretary of Health and Human Services as necessary to:

   A. Prevent healthcare fraud and abuse

   B. Ensure appropriate state regulation of insurance and health plans to the extent authorized by law

   C. Complete state reporting on healthcare delivery or costs

   D. Serve a compelling need related to public health, safety, or welfare, and the Secretary of Health and Human Services determines the privacy intrusion is warranted when balanced against the need

2. Regulates the manufacture, registration, distribution, dispensing or other control of any controlled substance as identified by federal or state law; or

3. Provides for the reporting of disease or injury, child abuse, birth, or death, or for the conduct of public health surveillance, investigation, or intervention; or

4. Requires a health plan to report or provide access to information for management or financial audits, program monitoring and evaluation, or licensure or certification of facilities or individuals

Source: 45 CFR 160.203

State laws vary in the amount of protection they give to patient information. Because of this, it has been necessary for states to perform preemption analyses. These analyses compare the HIPAA Privacy Rule with state laws to determine whether or not HIPAA preempts the state laws.

Public Health Reporting

All states have laws that require certain diseases or events to be reported. This information provides public health data that is beneficial for tracking the incidence and prevalence of diseases, tracking survival statistics, identifying high-risk populations, and trending many factors longitudinally.

Each state has its own child abuse and neglect statutes that mirror the federal **Child Abuse Prevention and Treatment Act (CAPTA) of 1996**. In general, there are four types of maltreatment: neglect, physical abuse, sexual abuse, and emotional abuse (Child Welfare Information Gateway 2010). For reporting purposes, children are generally defined as any person under the age of 18 or, if there is a physical or mental handicap, up to age 21. Those most commonly required to report suspected child abuse and neglect include healthcare practitioners, police officers, educators, and human service workers. State law may specify that an abused or neglected child's health information must be disclosed without authorization as part of an investigation. The disclosure does not violate the HIPAA Privacy Rule, and the state law that requires disclosure is not preempted by HIPAA, because of exceptions built into HIPAA. These exceptions are "required by law," "public health activities," or "disclosures about victims of abuse, neglect, or domestic violence" (Brodnik et al. 2012).

State laws also provide for mandatory reporting of suspected abuse of the elderly and disabled. Abuse of the elderly and disabled can be of several types including physical, emotional, financial, and sexual abuse; exploitation; neglect; and abandonment. State law may specify that an abused elderly or disabled person's health information must be disclosed without authorization as part of an investigation. The disclosure does not violate the HIPAA Privacy Rule and the state law that requires disclosure is not preempted by HIPAA because of exceptions built into HIPAA. These exceptions are "required by law" or "disclosures about victims of abuse, neglect, or domestic violence" (Brodnik et al. 2012).

Vital records document medical events such as births, deaths, abortions, and fetal deaths. Information is submitted by healthcare providers and others to local health departments and state vital statistics departments. They, in turn, are required to provide information to the **National Center for Health Statistics (NCHS)**, an agency within HHS, to compile this data nationally. Statistics that are generated as a result include birth and death rates, common causes of death, and common types of birth defects. State laws requiring the reporting of vital statistics without authorization do not violate the HIPAA Privacy Rule, and the state law that requires reporting is not preempted by HIPAA, because of the "public health activities" exception built into HIPAA (Brodnik et al. 2012).

Public health reporting also includes communicable diseases, which are transmitted through direct or indirect contact. State laws identify those diseases that must be reported in order to track and control outbreaks. Those most often required to report communicable diseases include an individual's attending physician or a person responsible for a hospital, emergency room, or other healthcare entity that is treating the individual. State law may provide that the information, although it must be reported, will remain confidential upon receipt. State laws requiring the reporting of communicable diseases do not violate the HIPAA Privacy Rule, and state laws that require reporting are not preempted by HIPAA because of the "public health activities" exception built into HIPAA. Further, in specific situations, HIPAA allows a covered entity to disclose health information to individuals that may be at risk of contracting or spreading a communicable disease (Brodnik et al. 2012). The HIPAA exceptions relevant to child abuse, abuse of the elderly and disabled, vital statistics, and public health reporting will be discussed further in chapter 3.

In addition to these events listed, other events that commonly must be reported per state law include unnatural deaths such as accidents, homicides, suicides, sudden deaths, and other suspicious deaths. Additionally, wounds such as burns and those inflicted by knife or gunshot often must be reported. Finally, national initiatives are in place to enhance systematic reporting of other unusual events such as medical errors (Brodnik et al. 2012).

CHECK YOUR UNDERSTANDING 1.1

Instructions: Indicate whether the following statements are true or false (T or F).

1. The Freedom of Information Act requires disclosure of health records.
2. The HITECH Act of ARRA of 2009 made changes to the HIPAA Privacy Rule.
3. Preemption requires compliance with state law when a federal law and state law conflict with one another.
4. Drug and alcohol abuse treatment records received protection under federal law prior to the HIPAA Privacy Rule.
5. The Conditions of Participation regulate providers who receive funds from the Medicare and Medicaid programs.

Section 3: Accrediting and Certifying Bodies

Accreditation Organizations

Accreditation is a voluntary process that an organization undergoes to establish credibility and status as a member of its industry. It is a determination by an external body that an organization has achieved predefined standards established by that body (Gregg Fahrenholz 2012). Accreditation is obtained through a number of assessments including on-site surveys, documentation reviews, and scrutiny of an organization's processes. A type of "gold standard," accreditation permits a healthcare organization to announce itself as meeting or exceeding the highest level of performance and patient care. In addition to this recognition, however, accreditation also offers a number of other benefits. They are outlined in figure 1.2.

In the context of accreditation, healthcare providers also have certification options. **Certification** by an accreditation organization is generally limited to a particular program, such as certification of asthma, heart failure, and diabetes programs. Aside from accreditation organizations, certification can also apply to entire organizations, such as Medicare-certified hospices, and individuals (for example, the Registered Health Information Administrator [RHIA] designation is a certification). As described later in

FIGURE 1.2. Benefits of accreditation

- Attracts patients, professional staff, and third-party payers
- Enhances reputation and community confidence by demonstrating a commitment to excellence
- Enables organizations to meet certain regulatory agency certification and state licensure requirements in an alternative manner
- Provides a report card of the quality of an organization's performance
- Serves as an educational tool and enables continuous performance improvement

Source: Gregg Fahrenholz 2011

this section, certification also applies to EHR products that federal government designees have recognized as possessing required characteristics.

There are several bodies that accredit healthcare organizations. The ones that will be discussed in this chapter are the Joint Commission, American Osteopathic Association (AOA), Accreditation Association for Ambulatory Health Care (AAAHC), Commission on Accreditation of Rehabilitation Facilities (CARF), and National Committee for Quality Assurance (NCQA). The protection of health information is an important part of these organizations' accreditation standards.

The Joint Commission

The **Joint Commission** is the oldest and most recognized healthcare accrediting body. Its predecessor was established by the American College of Surgeons in 1917 as a hospital inspection program. As a collaborative effort among several organizations, it became known as The Joint Commission on the Accreditation of Hospitals (JCAH) in 1951. As its scope changed and it accredited more than just hospitals, its name changed as well. It was renamed The Joint Commission on the Accreditation of Healthcare Organizations (JCAHO) in 1987. It is now simply called the Joint Commission and it accredits healthcare organizations in many service areas (Gregg Fahrenholz 2012). Many healthcare organizations seek Joint Commission accreditation because its standards represent accepted practice related to quality patient care (Joint Commission 2012). The Joint Commission has deeming authority by the **Centers for Medicare and Medicaid Services (CMS)** to survey for compliance with the CoP. If an organization meets the Joint Commission's standards, CMS will deem the organization to have also met the CoP. The service areas that the Joint Commission accredits are outlined in figure 1.3.

The format of the Joint Commission's expectations has changed over time, but its standards define performance expectations necessary for a safe and high-quality treatment setting (Joint Commission 2012). Standards related to health information reside in two chapters: Information Management and Record of Care, Treatment, and Services. Each chapter contains a series of standards that are detailed by specific elements of performance (Gregg Fahrenholz 2012). The standards pertaining to the privacy and security of health information reside in the Information Management chapter and state that "the hospital protects the privacy of health information" (IM 02.01.01) and "the hospital maintains the security and integrity of health information" (IM 02.01.03) (Joint Commission 2011).

FIGURE 1.3.	Service areas accredited by the Joint Commission

Ambulatory health care
Behavioral health care
Critical access hospitals
Home care
Hospitals
Laboratory services
Long-term care

Source: Joint Commission 2012

FIGURE 1.4.	Service areas accredited by the American Osteopathic Association (AOA)

Acute care
Ambulatory care or office-based surgery
Ambulatory surgical centers
Behavioral and mental health
Clinical laboratories
Critical access hospitals
Primary stroke centers

Source: AOA 2012

American Osteopathic Association

The **American Osteopathic Association (AOA)** represents osteopathic physicians and accredits osteopathic medical schools and training programs. It has also been a healthcare organization accrediting body since 1945. It accredits hospitals and other healthcare facilities through its **Healthcare Facilities Accreditation Program (HFAP)**. The AOA has deeming authority by the Centers for Medicare and Medicaid Services to survey for compliance with the CoP (AOA 2012). If an organization meets the AOA's HFAP standards, which are closely aligned with the CoP, CMS will deem the organization to have also met the CoP. The AOA accredits many service areas, as outlined in figure 1.4.

Accreditation Association for Ambulatory Health Care

The **Accreditation Association for Ambulatory Health Care (AAAHC)**, also called the Accreditation Association, was formed in 1979. Its focus is on all aspects of ambulatory healthcare organizations (AAAHC 2012). In states such as Florida and California, AAAHC accreditation is accepted as compliance with specific state laws. Medicare deemed status has been granted to ambulatory surgery centers and managed care organizations (through the Medicare Advantage program) that are AAAHC accredited (Gregg Fahrenholz 2012). The service areas that the AAAHC accredits are outlined in figure 1.5.

Commission on Accreditation of Rehabilitation Facilities

The **Commission on Accreditation of Rehabilitation Facilities (CARF)** was formed in 1966 as a merger between the Association of Rehabilitation Centers and the National Association of Sheltered Workshops and Homebound Programs. It focuses on health and human service providers and has an international scope (CARF 2012). The service areas that CARF accredits are listed in figure 1.6.

National Committee for Quality Assurance

The **National Committee for Quality Assurance (NCQA)** was founded in 1990 and began accrediting managed care organizations such as health maintenance organizations (HMOs), preferred provide organizations (PPOs), and consumer-directed health plans in 1991 (NCQA 2012). It is most recognized for accrediting health plans, but it also accredits many types of healthcare organizations. Regarding health plan accreditation, many large employers only offer health plans to their employees that are NCQA-accredited. Further,

FIGURE 1.5.	Service areas accredited by the Accreditation Association for Ambulatory Health Care (AAAHC)

Ambulatory healthcare clinics
Ambulatory surgery centers
Birthing centers
College and university health centers
Community health centers
Dental group practices
Diagnostic imaging centers
Endoscopy centers
Federally qualified community health centers
Health maintenance organizations (HMOs)
Independent physician associations (IPAs)
Indian health centers
Lithotripsy centers
Managed care organizations
Medical home organizations
Military healthcare facilities
Multi-specialty group practices
Occupational health centers
Office-based anesthesia organizations
Office-based surgery centers and practices
Oral and maxillofacial surgeons' offices
Pain management centers
Podiatry practices
Radiation oncology centers
Single–specialty group practices
Surgical recovery centers
Urgent or immediate care centers
Women's health centers

Source: AAAHC 2012

FIGURE 1.6.	Service areas accredited by the Commission on Accreditation of Rehabilitation Facilities (CARF)

Aging services
Behavioral health
Business and services management networks
Child and youth services
Durable medical equipment, prosthetics, orthotics, and supplies
Employment and community services
Medical rehabilitation
Opiod treatment programs
Vision rehabilitation services

Source: CARF 2012

FIGURE 1.7.	Service areas accredited by the National Committee for Quality Assurance (NCQA)

Accountable care organizations
Health plan accreditation
Wellness and health promotion
Managed behavioral healthcare organizations
New health plans
Disease management

Source: NCQA 2012

more than 30 states exempt NCQA-accredited organizations from state audit requirements (NCQA 2012). The **Healthcare Effectiveness and Data Information Set (HEDIS)** is a tool offered by NCQA that measures the quality of health plans. Health plan purchasers—which are mostly employers—and consumers use it to compare health plan performances (Gregg Fahrenholz 2012). The service areas that NCQA accredits are listed in figure 1.7.

ONC-Authorized EHR Certification Bodies

The adoption of electronic health records (EHRs) among healthcare providers has been a continuous process. As this section will discuss, the federal government has propelled this process forward by creating guidelines and financial incentives for EHR adoption.

EHR Adoption and Meaningful Use

For several years the federal government has promoted the adoption of health information technology, specifically the EHR, by healthcare providers. The **Office of the National Coordinator for Health Information Technology (ONC)**, an agency within HHS, was formed in 2004 via presidential executive order to guide this initiative. The agency was later codified (established by statute) via ARRA. However, adopting an EHR has been daunting for many providers. The significant cost of adopting an EHR has been the greatest concern. There are also logistical concerns associated with implementing both a new product and a new workflow. Finally, many providers with little knowledge of technology have been overwhelmed with the prospect of selecting one EHR vendor from dozens of options. How do they discern good products from bad products, and reputable vendors from vendors that are not trustworthy or not likely to remain in business to provide technical supports and upgrades?

One of the most important steps a provider can take is to select an electronic health record that has been certified by an ONC-authorized technology review body. These ONC designees, **Office of the National Coordinator for Health Information Technology-Authorized Testing and Certification Bodies (ONC-ATCBs)** and **Office of the National Coordinator for Health Information Technology-Authorized Certification Bodies (ONC-ACBs)**, test EHR systems to make sure they comply with HHS standards and certification criteria. If they do, the EHR systems are certified. By purchasing a certified product, a provider is ensured that the EHR meets key standards and is capable of performing the required functions (ONC 2012). The ONC-ATCB program will sunset when the permanent ONC-ACB certification program is in place. This was to occur no earlier than January 1, 2012, and it has been delayed.

In addition to required privacy and security features, an important element of certification is **meaningful use**, which describes a government-prescribed level of effective EHR use. According to ARRA, "three components of meaningful use are: (1) use of a certified EHR in a meaningful manner, (2) use of certified EHR technology for electronic exchange of health information to improve quality of healthcare, and (3) use of certified EHR technology to submit clinical quality and other measures" (CMS 2012). Three meaningful use time periods have been established. Under Stage 1, hospitals must meet 14 required core objectives and must select five menu set objectives from 10 options to achieve meaningful use. Eligible professionals (including physicians, dentists, optometrists, chiropractors, and podiatrists) must meet 15 required core objectives and must select five menu set objectives from 10 options to achieve meaningful use. Figures 1.8 and 1.9 list the required core objectives and the menu set objectives for hospitals and eligible professionals, respectively. To be staged in over five years, Stage 1 (years 2011 and 2012) sets meaningful use baseline criteria. Stage 2 (with the final administrative rule published in August 2012) and Stage 3 (expected for year 2015) will expand on the baseline criteria (CMS 2012). Without providing functionalities that enable a hospital or eligible provider to meet meaningful use criteria, an EHR product cannot be certified. Although the ultimate goal of EHR use is improved patient care, Stage 1 is designed primarily to motivate providers to implement EHRs (Dimick 2011). Elements of Stage 2 include:

- "Allowing patients to view online, download, and transmit their health information from participating physicians within four business days of the information being available"

- Requiring eligible hospitals to "allow patients the ability to view online, download, and transmit their health information within 36 hours of discharge"

- Requiring physicians and hospital staff to "track how many patients access their health records during the program reporting period" (to meet meaningful use requirements, greater than five percent of patients seen by a physician or discharged by a hospital must access their records)

- Requiring healthcare providers to "offer and use secure electronic messaging to communicate with patients on relevant health information" (to meet meaningful use requirements, five percent of patients must use this feature)

- Aligning "clinical quality measures with other reporting programs to reduce burden and duplication of efforts" and

- Transitioning "all HIT Menu Set measures to Core Set of measures except for electronic syndromic surveillance data and advance directives"

FIGURE 1.8.	Hospital core objectives and menu set objectives for Stage 1 meaningful use
Core Objectives	
1	Use computerized provider order entry (CPOE) for medication orders directly entered by any licensed healthcare professional who can enter orders into the medical record per state, local, and professional guidelines.
2	Implement drug–drug and drug–allergy interaction checks.

(Continued on next page)

FIGURE 1.8.	(Continued)

	Core Objectives
3	Maintain an up-to-date problem list of current and active diagnoses.
4	Maintain active medication list.
5	Maintain active medication allergy list.
6	Record all of the following demographics: preferred language; gender; race; ethnicity; date of birth; date and preliminary cause of death in the event of mortality in the eligible hospital or critical access hospital.
7	Record and chart changes in the following vital signs: height; weight; blood pressure; calculate and display body mass index (BMI); plot and display growth charts for children 2 to 20 years, including BMI.
8	Record smoking for patients 13 years old or older.
9	Report hospital clinical quality measures to CMS or, in the case of Medicaid eligible hospitals, the states.
10	Implement on clinical decision support rule related to a high priority hospital condition along with the ability to track compliance with that rule.
11	Provide patients with an electronic copy of their health information (including diagnostic tests results, problem list, medication lists, medication allergies, discharge summary, procedures), upon request.
12	Provide patients with an electronic copy of their discharge instructions at time of discharge, upon request.
13	Capability to exchange key clinical information (for example, problem list, medication list, medication allergies, and diagnostic test results), among providers of care and patient authorized entities electronically.
14	Protect electronic health information created or maintained by the certified EHR technology through the implementation of appropriate technical capabilities.

	Menu Set Objectives
1	Implement drug formulary checks.
2	Record advance directives for patients 64 years old or older.
3	Incorporate clinical lab-test results into EHR as structured data.
4	Generate lists of patients by specific conditions to use for quality improvement, reduction of disparities, research, or outreach.
5	Use certified EHR technology to identify patient-specific education resources and provide those resources to the patient if appropriate.

FIGURE 1.8.	(Continued)
	Menu Set Objectives
6	The eligible hospital or critical access hospital that receives a patient from another setting of care or provider of care or believes an encounter is relevant should perform medication reconciliation.
7	The eligible hospital or critical access hospital that transitions their patient to another setting of care or provider of care or refers their patient to another provider of care should provide summary care record for each transition of care or referral.
8	Capability to submit electronic data to immunization registries or immunization information systems and actual submission according to applicable law and practice.
9	Capability to submit electronic data on reportable (as required by state or local law) lab results to public health agencies and actual submission according to applicable law and practice.
10	Capability to submit electronic syndromic surveillance data to public health agencies and actual submission according to applicable law and practice.

Source: CMS 2012

FIGURE 1.9.	Eligible professional core objectives and menu set objectives for Stage 1 meaningful use
	Core Objectives
1	Use computerized provider order entry (CPOE) for medication orders directly entered by any licensed healthcare professional who can enter orders into the medical record per state, local, and professional guidelines.
2	Implement drug–drug and drug–allergy interaction checks.
3	Maintain an up-to-date problem list of current and active diagnoses.
4	Generate and transmit permissible prescriptions electronically (eRx).
5	Maintain active medication list.
6	Maintain active medication allergy list.
7	Record all of the following demographics: preferred language; gender; race; ethnicity; date of birth.

(*Continued on next page*)

FIGURE 1.9.	(Continued)
8	Record and chart changes in the following vital signs: height; weight; blood pressure; calculate and display body mass index (BMI); plot and display growth charts for children 2 to 20 years, including BMI.
9	Record smoking status for patients 13 years old or older.
10	Report ambulatory clinical quality measures to CMS or, in the case of Medicaid eligible professionals, the states.
11	Implement on clinical decision support rule relevant to specialty or high clinical priority along with the ability to track compliance with that rule.
12	Provide patients with an electronic copy of their health information (including diagnostic tests results, problem list, medication lists, medication allergies) upon request.
13	Provide clinical summaries for patients for each office visit.
14	Capability to exchange key clinical information (for example, problem list, medication list, allergies, and diagnostic test results), among providers of care and patient authorized entities electronically.
15	Protect electronic health information created or maintained by the certified EHR technology through the implementation of appropriate technical capabilities.
	Menu Set Objectives
1	Implement drug formulary checks.
2	Incorporate clinical lab-test results into EHR as structured data.
3	Generate lists of patients by specific conditions to use for quality improvement, reduction of disparities, research, or outreach.
4	Send patient reminders per patient preference for preventive or follow-up care.
5	Provide patients with timely electronic access to their health information (including lab results, problem list, medication lists, and allergies) within four business days of the information being available to the eligible professional.
6	Use certified EHR technology to identify patient-specific education resources and provide those resources to the patient if appropriate.
7	The eligible professional who receives a patient from another setting of care or provider of care or believes an encounter is relevant should perform medication reconciliation.
8	The eligible professional who transitions their patient to another setting of care or provider of care or refers their patient to another provider of care should provide summary care record for each transition of care or referral.

FIGURE 1.9.	(Continued)
Menu Set Objectives	
9	Capability to submit electronic data to immunization registries or immunization information systems and actual submission according to applicable law and practice.
10	Capability to submit electronic syndromic surveillance data to public health agencies and actual submission according to applicable law and practice.

Source: CMS 2012

FIGURE 1.10.	Description of EHR adoption incentive plan timelines for eligible professionals				
	Qualifies to Receive First Medicare Incentive Payment in ...				
Payment Amount by Year	**2011**	**2012**	**2013**	**2014**	**2015**
2011	$18,000	–	–	–	–
2012	$12,000	$18,000	–	–	–
2013	$8,000	$12,000	$15,000	–	–
2014	$4,000	$8,000	$12,000	$12,000	–
2015	$2,000	$4,000	$8,000	$8,000	–
2016	-	$2,000	$4,000	$4,000	–
Total payment	$44,000	$44,000	$39,000	$24,000	–

Source: Dimick 2011

The compliance date for Stage 2 meaningful use is 2014. (AHIMA 2012)

Payments from the federal government have already begun for those who have demonstrated Stage 1 meaningful use. Eligible professionals in the Medicare EHR Incentive Program must achieve meaningful use of a certified product by 2014 to be eligible to receive the government's incentive payments. Funds for incentive payments were established in ARRA. A final rule by CMS in July 2010 established the details of the incentive program, which was developed in conjunction with ONC. The first EHR products were certified for the incentive programs in autumn 2010. Registration for the Medicare program began in January 2011. For demonstrating meaningful use of certified health IT systems, physicians in the Medicare program are eligible to earn up to $44,000. If they qualify for the first payment in 2011 or 2012, they can receive the full amount. The meaningful use incentive plan timeline for eligible professionals is detailed in figure 1.10. It shows that providers who enter the incentive program early earn the greatest amount of money (Dimick 2011).

Hospitals are also eligible to receive incentives for implementing and using certified EHR technology. Hospital earnings can run well into the millions of dollars, with a base payment of $2 million and additional payments based on the number of discharges within a payment year (CMS 2012). Hospitals that do not qualify for payments until 2014 or 2015 will receive reduced incentive payments. After 2015, hospital incentive payments will no longer be available. In 2015, physicians face monetary penalties in the form of reduced reimbursements for non-adoption or failure to demonstrate meaningful use (Dimick 2011).

The Medicaid EHR Incentive Program, which is not available in all states, operates somewhat differently. Year 2016 is the deadline for eligible providers to adopt an EHR and qualify for their first payment, but annual payments do not diminish for eligible professionals who delay implementation. Payment in the first year is $21,250 and $8,500 in each subsequent year. The Medicaid program does not issue penalties. Eligible hospitals may begin receiving payments any fiscal year between 2011 and 2016 (Dimick 2011).

Certification Commission for Health Information Technology

There are now several organizations that have been authorized by ONC to test and certify EHR systems. However, the **Certification Commission for Health Information Technology (CCHIT)** is the oldest ONC-authorized EHR certification body. It was created in 2004 and has certified EHRs since 2006. It tests systems for "integrated functionality, interoperability, and security" (CCHIT 2012). The CCHIT is an ONC-ATCB, described more fully in the next section.

Other ONC-ATCBs and ONC-ACBs

The ONC certification process, developed to make sure that EHR products meet adopted standards, certification criteria, and other technical requirements to achieve meaningful use, has evolved. Originally carried out by CCHIT, eventually the ONC-ATCB and ONC-ACB programs were developed.

In the ONC-ATCB program, which is temporary, ONC-ATCBs are authorized by the ONC to test and certify EHR technology. The ONC acts as the accrediting body for the ONC-ATCBs. The program includes certification of both complete EHRs and EHR modules. The temporary ONC-ATCB program was created to ensure providers had certified EHRs in place, which is required to pursue meaningful use incentives. Per HITECH, only certifications issued by an ONC-ATCB are considered to have met the "Certified EHR Technology" requirement necessary to quality for Medicare and Medicaid EHR incentive payment programs. ONC-ATCBs are

- Surescripts LLC
- ICSA Labs
- SLI Global Solutions
- InfoGard Laboratories, Inc.
- CCHIT
- Drummond Group, Inc. (ONC 2012)

The permanent ONC-ACB certification program will replace the ONC-ATCB program. For testing, the **National Institute of Standards and Technology (NIST) National Voluntary Laboratory Accreditation Program (NVLAP)** will be the ONC-AA **(Office of the National Coordinator for Health Information Technology-Approved Accreditor)** that accredits organizations to test EHR technology. The **American National Standards Institute (ANSI)** will serve as the certification accreditor, with re-application to occur after three years. ONC-ATCBs do not automatically become ONC-ACBs, but apply for the designation. The ONC-ACB designation must be renewed every three years (ONC 2012). In July 2012, ANSI accredited five organizations that may apply to ONC for certification status in the permanent program. NVLAP also accredited five programs to serve as Accredited Testing Laboratories (ATLs) and test EHR technology under the permanent program. The certification and testing programs are separate processes and must be completed independently of each other by organizations that have been designed as both ONC-ACBs and ATLs. The five organizations accredited as certification bodies are

1. CCHIT
2. Drummond Group, Inc.
3. ICSA Labs
4. InfoGard Laboratories, Inc.
5. Orion Register, Inc.

The five organizations accredited as ATLs are

1. CCHIT
2. Drummond Group, Inc.
3. ICSA Labs
4. InfoGard Laboratories, Inc.
5. SLI Global Solutions (ONC 2012)

Electronic Healthcare Network Accreditation Commission

The **Electronic Healthcare Network Accreditation Commission (EHNAC)** was formed in 1993. Recognized by the federal government, it accredits electronic health networks by assessing them against electronic transaction standards. The organization's three accreditation options are the Healthcare Network Accreditation Program (HNAP) for organizations managing and transferring protected health information; the Financial Services Accreditation Program (FSAP) for banks, financial services firms and vendors; and the e-Prescribing Accreditation Program (ePAP), which assesses an organization's electronic prescribing and fax-based prescribing transactions for factors including security and timeliness, and conformance to industry-standard formats. As with all other accreditations, organizations that are accredited by EHNAC do so for promotional purposes and to demonstrate compliance with industry standards (EHNAC 2012).

Section 4: Professional Ethical Standards and Codes of Conduct

Ethical standards and codes of conduct govern a variety of healthcare professions, including the health information management profession. The **American Health Information Management Association (AHIMA) Code of Ethics** has guided the protection of patient information for several decades. Revised in 2011, it states that health information management professionals "preserve, protect, and secure personal health information in any form or medium and hold in the highest regards health information and other information of a confidential nature..." (AHIMA 2011). Although the AHIMA Code of Ethics does not have the force of law, its ethical principles provide guidance to members of the profession (Brodnik et al. 2012). It is evidence of a credentialed individual's professional values and principles. It is also binding for all AHIMA members and those who hold an AHIMA credential (AHIMA 2011). Violation of the Code of Ethics can result in disciplinary action including revocation of one's AHIMA credential.

Section 5: Organizational Policy

An organization's internal policies are extremely important. Like professional ethical standards and codes of conduct, they do not have the force of law. Nonetheless, they play an important legal role. Policies are evidence of an organization's mission and values. Further it is important that an organization trains all workforce members on its policies and ensures they are enforced. These actions demonstrate the organization's commitment to stay true to its mission and values. Once developed, failure to enforce or comply with policies can result in liability for both an organization and its employees.

CHECK YOUR UNDERSTANDING 1.2

Instructions: Indicate whether the following statements are true or false (T or F).

1. The Joint Commission's HFAP accreditation standards are closely aligned with the Medicare Conditions of Participation.
2. Health plans may be accredited by the National Committee for Quality Assurance (NCQA).
3. Demonstration of meaningful use of a certified EHR product may result in incentive payments from the federal government.
4. The ONC-ACB program will sunset, to be replaced by the permanent ONC-ATCB certification program.
5. A profession's Code of Ethics has the force of law.

REAL-WORLD CASE

Under the EHR incentive payment program for meaningful use, providers in the best position are those who were already undergoing EHR implementation when the incentive program began. Because of their more numerous resources and more complex governance and infrastructure, larger hospitals operate on a bigger scale. This puts them at a distinct advantage over smaller hospitals and private physician practices. Further, hospital systems running a single enterprise EHR platform have an advantage over providers with a variety of interfaced systems where upgrades may be necessary and staff will have to be retrained before Stage 1 meaningful use measures can be attempted (Dimick 2011).

Even with these advantages, however, incentives paid to major EHR users do not cover costs associated with installing the system. For example, NorthShore University HealthSystem, based in Evanston, IL, first implemented an EHR in 2003. After reporting its Stage 1 meaningful use measures it received its first incentive payment of $8 million. This amount, plus additional incentive payments, will still not cover the organization's total IT investment, which the organization estimates as well above $100 million. However, for many hospitals the incentive program was not the driving factor behind EHR implementation. It was improved patient care. The gap between incentive payments and investment costs may be less for small physician offices because their overhead is lower and they will be implementing smaller EHR systems (Dimick 2011).

SUMMARY

Health information is regulated in many different ways. Laws governing health information are generally viewed as having the greatest force and effect. However, accreditation and certification standards, professional codes of ethics, and internal organizational policies are also compelling. From this chapter, the reader should understand that *all* of these regulatory mechanisms need to be consulted when accessing, using, or disclosing health information.

REFERENCES

Accreditation Association for Ambulatory Health Care. 2012. http://www.aaahc.org.

American Health Information Management Association. 2012. Stage 2 Meaningful Use Final Rule Released. *Journal of AHIMA*. http://journal.ahima.org/2012/08/23/stage-2-meaningful-use-final-rule-released/.

American Health Information Management Association. 2011. Code of Ethics. http://library.ahima.org/xpedio/groups/public/documents/ahima/bok1_024277.hcsp?dDocName=bok1_024277.

American Osteopathic Association. 2012. http://www.aoa.org.

Brodnik, M., R. Reynolds, and L. Rinehart-Thompson. 2012. *Fundamentals of Law for Health Informatics and Information Management*. Chicago: AHIMA.

Centers for Medicare and Medicaid Services. 2012. https://www.cms.gov/.

Certification Commission for Health Information Technology. 2012. http://www.cchit.org/about.

Child Welfare Information Gateway. 2010. http://www.childwelfare.gov/.

Commission on Accreditation of Rehabilitation Facilities. 2012. http://www.carf.org.

Department of Health and Human Services. 2010. http://www.hhs.gov/.

Dimick, C. 2011. Meaningful use: Notes from the journey. *Journal of AHIMA* 82(10): 24–30.

Electronic Healthcare Network Accreditation Commission. 2012. http://www.ehnac.org/.

Gregg Fahrenholz, Cheryl. 2011. *Documentation for Medical Practices.* Chicago: AHIMA.

Joint Commission. 2011. *Comprehensive Accreditation Manual for Hospitals.* Oakbrook Terrace, IL: Joint Commission.

Joint Commission. 2012. http://www.thejointcommission.org.

National Committee for Quality Assurance. 2012. http://www.ncqa.org.

Office of the National Coordinator for Health Information Technology. 2012. http://healthit.hhs.gov/.

45 CFR Part 160 Subpart B: Preemption of State Law. 2006.

45 CFR 160.203: General rule and exceptions. 2006.

5 USC §552: Freedom of information act of 1967.

CHAPTER 2

HIPAA Privacy and Security: The Basics

Learning Objectives

- Explain the HIPAA statute and administrative rules

- Discuss the scope of HIPAA and the purposes it serves in addition to protecting patient information

- Identify to whom and to what HIPAA applies

- Define and describe HIPAA terms of art and explain why they are important

- Describe the various types of organizations governed by HIPAA

KEY TERMS

Administrative simplification	Individual
Affiliated covered entity	Legal health record (LHR)
Business associate (BA)	Limited data set
Business associate agreement (BAA)	Minimum necessary
Covered entity	Organized healthcare arrangement
Data use agreement	Payment
Deidentified information	Personal representative
Designated record set (DRS)	Privacy
Disclosure	Protected health information
Health plan	Request
Healthcare clearinghouse	Security
Healthcare operations	Shadow records
Healthcare provider	Treatment
Hybrid entity	Treatment, Payment, and Operations (TPO)
Hybrid health record	Use
In loco parentis	Workforce

INTRODUCTION

Before discussing HIPAA's many requirements and exceptions, one should first be familiar with the scope of privacy and security in the context of the HIPAA statute; the types of individuals and organizations that must comply with HIPAA; and information that is and is not protected by HIPAA. These concepts will be covered in this chapter, along with a number of other relevant terms and provisions.

Section 1: Privacy and Security in the HIPAA Statute

Privacy, as it relates to one's health information, is the right of a patient to control disclosure of that information (AHIMA 2012). **Security**, as it relates to one's health information, refers to measures that control access and protect information from unauthorized disclosure, alteration, destruction or loss while maintaining availability for those who need it (AHIMA 2012). The HIPAA security rule requires those who are bound by it to

- Ensure confidentiality, integrity, and availability of all electronic protected health information created, received, maintained, or transmitted
- Protect against reasonably anticipated threats or hazards that might affect the security of integrity of electronic protected health information

- Protect against reasonably anticipated uses or disclosures of electronic protected health information that is not permitted or required
- Ensure workforce compliance (45 CFR 164.306(a))

The security rule and its requirements related to electronic protected health information will be discussed in greater detail in chapter 4.

Whereas privacy focuses on the rights of an individual with regard to his or her information, security focuses on how to safeguard the information. Although there is a clear distinction between the two concepts, many of the terms and principles introduced in this chapter are common to both HIPAA privacy and HIPAA security.

HIPAA was enacted by Congress in 1996 and stands for the Health Insurance Portability and Accountability Act. HIPAA amended three pieces of federal legislation that already existed: the Internal Revenue Code of 1986, the Employee Retirement Income Security Act of 1986 (ERISA), and the Public Health Service Act (Brodnik et al. 2012).

When people hear the acronym HIPAA, they most likely think first of health information privacy because that is what has received the greatest amount of media attention. However, the HIPAA statute encompasses more than just patient privacy. HIPAA consists of five broad sections, which are called titles. Most of the titles do not address the protection of patient information. Figure 2.1 displays the five titles of the HIPAA statute. As the figure shows, Title II contains privacy and security.

| FIGURE 2.1. | The five titles of the HIPAA Statute |

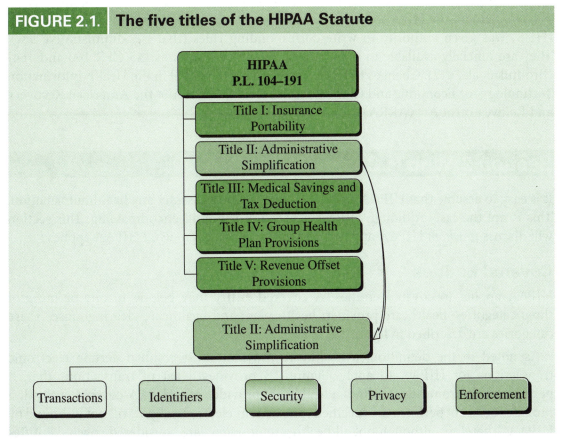

Source: Walsh 2011

Title I, portability, allows for the continuation of health insurance coverage and protects individuals and their dependents from losing coverage when they leave or otherwise change jobs. This title also prohibits discrimination based on a person's status or his dependents' status when he enrolls in a health insurance plan or is charged health insurance premiums.

Title II includes provisions about healthcare fraud and abuse prevention and medical liability (medical malpractice) reform. For purposes of this book, the portion of Title II that deals with administrative simplification is the most important. This is because both the privacy and security rules reside there, as does the enforcement rule. The administrative simplification portion of Title II also addresses transactions and code set standardization requirements and unique national provider identifiers that are beyond the scope of this book. **Administrative simplification** is HIPAA's effort to standardize the healthcare industry's nonuniform and inefficient business practices (for example, billing), many of which involve electronic data transmission. Concerns about the protection of electronic health information led to the subsequent creation of the HIPAA privacy and security rules (Brodnik et al. 2012).

Titles III, IV, and V pertain to the Internal Revenue Code, include tax-related provisions, and also contain group health plan requirements. Title III specifically provides deductions for medical insurance. Title IV addresses group health plan coverage for individuals who have pre-existing conditions and also includes income tax requirements for specific groups (Brodnik et al. 2012).

To implement the HIPAA statute, the US Department of Health and Human Services (HHS) was given authority to write corresponding rules (that is, administrative law). They are officially available in the Code of Federal Regulations (45 CFR 160 and 164) (Brodnik et al. 2012). Changes to HIPAA were enacted in 2009 in the Health Information Technology for Economic and Clinical Health (HITECH) Act of the American Recovery and Reinvestment Act (ARRA).

Section 2: Who Is Covered by HIPAA

It is easy to assume that HIPAA applies to anyone who possesses any health information. This is not the case. Although HIPAA is broad, it is not all-encompassing. This section will discuss *to whom* HIPAA applies. Section 3 will discuss *to what* HIPAA applies.

Covered Entities

HIPAA applies to covered entities. A **covered entity** may belong to one or more of three categories: healthcare provider; health plan; and healthcare clearinghouse. These categories are described in figure 2.2.

As noted in the definition, a healthcare provider must conduct certain electronic transactions for HIPAA to apply. Figure 2.3 provides a list of transactions that, if performed electronically, qualifies a healthcare provider as a HIPAA-covered entity. If a provider does not perform the specified transactions electronically, it will not be bound by HIPAA. Therefore, although not all healthcare providers are considered covered entities by definition, those not covered by HIPAA constitute a small percentage.

FIGURE 2.2.	HIPAA covered entities

A **healthcare provider** who transmits any health information pertaining to certain transactions (financial or administrative) in electronic form. A healthcare provider can range from an individual practitioner to a large healthcare organization.

A **health plan**, which is an individual or group plan that provides or pays the costs of medical care.

A **healthcare clearinghouse**, which is an entity that process billing transactions between a healthcare provider and a health plan.

Source: 45 CFR 160.103

FIGURE 2.3.	Electronic transactions by HIPAA-covered healthcare providers

Health claims or equivalent encounter information
Enrollment and disenrollment in a health plan
Eligibility for a health plan
Health care payment and remittance advice
Health plan premium payments
Health care claim status
Referral certification and authorization
Coordination of benefits
First report of injury
Health claims attachments
Other transactions prescribed by the Secretary of HHS

Source: 45 CFR 160.103

Business Associates

In addition to covered entities, business associates must also comply with the HIPAA privacy and security rules. HIPAA has always addressed business associates. However, as described here, business associates now face much more stringent obligations and penalties for noncompliance per the HITECH changes to HIPAA.

Identifying Business Associates

A **business associate** (BA) is a person or organization, not a part of a covered entity's workforce, that performs functions or activities on behalf of or affecting a covered entity that involves the use or disclosure of individually identifiable health information (45 CFR 160.103(1)). The concept of individually identifiable health information will be introduced later in the chapter. BAs include organizations such as billing and consulting companies, accounting firms, and law firms that provide outside legal counsel to a covered entity (Brodnik et al. 2012). BAs also include persons such as individual consultants and individuals who operate their own transcription service. The common factor is that the person or organization performs services for the covered entity that involve health information.

Business Associate Agreements

Under HIPAA as it was originally written, BAs became legally obligated as BAs once they were associated with a covered entity and identified as a BA through a contract called a **business associate agreement** (BAA). The legal theory under which BAs are bound by HIPAA changed under HITECH. In general, as HIPAA requirements are explained throughout the chapter, it is understood that they also apply to BAs.

Once a covered entity identifies a person or organization as a BA, it is the covered entity's responsibility to initiate a BAA. This document legally protects patient information that is handled outside the covered entity on behalf of the covered entity. The written and signed BAA permits covered entities to lawfully disclose protected health information (PHI) to BAs. In the BAA, the BA agrees to the provider's requirements to use and disclose PHI only in ways that will protect the information's security and confidentiality. It also agrees to protect patient information from unauthorized access, use, or disclosure (Brodnik et al. 2012).

Figure 2.4 outlines the elements that a BAA between a covered entity and its BA should contain, including HITECH's requirements.

FIGURE 2.4. | **Elements of a business associate contract**

The requirements placed on business associates under HIPAA and ensuing HITECH legislation have heightened the importance of business associate agreements. Covered entities cannot disclose PHI to business associates unless the two have entered into a written contract that meets HIPAA and HITECH requirements. Under HITECH, privacy, security, and breach notification requirements apply to business associates.

Such a contract would include provisions that

- Prohibit the business associate from using or disclosing the PHI for any purpose other than that stated in the contract, and pursuant to the Privacy Rule and minimum necessary standard
- Prohibit the business associate from using or disclosing the PHI in a manner that would violate the requirements of the HIPAA Privacy Rule
- Require the business associate to maintain safeguards, as necessary, to ensure that the PHI is not used or disclosed except as provided by the contract
- Require the business associate to report to the covered entity any use or disclosure of the PHI that is not provided for in the contract
- Clarify that the business associate is responsible to report breaches of unsecured PHI
- Clarify that the business associate must adhere to policy and procedure, and documentation requirements imposed by the HIPAA Security Rule
- Establish how the covered entity would provide access to PHI to the individual whom the information is about when the business associate has made any material alterations to the information

FIGURE 2.4. **(Continued)**

- Require the business associate to make available its internal practices, books, and records relating to the use and disclosure of PHI received from the covered entity to the Department of Health and Human Services or its agents
- Establish how the entity would provide access to PHI to the individual whom the information is about in circumstances where the business associate holds the information and the covered entity does not
- Require the business associate to incorporate any amendments or corrections to the PHI when notified by the covered entity that the information is inaccurate or incomplete
- At termination of the contract, require the business associate to return or destroy all PHI received from the covered entity that it still maintains and prohibit the associate from retaining it
- State that individuals who are the subject of disclosed PHI are intended third-party beneficiaries of the contract
- Authorize the covered entity to terminate the contract when it determines that the business associate has repeatedly violated a term required in the contract
- State the business associate is subject to the HIPAA Security Rule, including implementation of administrative, technical, and procedural safeguards, and procedural and documentation requirements
- State that the business associate will receive satisfactory assurances from its subcontractors that the subcontractors will appropriately safeguard protected health information
- State that subcontractors of the business associate are responsible for complying with HIPAA and are directly liable for HIPAA violations, as is the business associate, even if the business associate has not entered into a contractual agreement with the subcontractor
- Clarify that the business associate is responsible to take action, possibly including termination, against a subcontractor if it violates HIPAA or provisions of the BAA
- Clarify that the business associate is subject to civil monetary penalties for violation of the Privacy Rule or the Security Rule

Source: Adapted from Cassidy 2000; updated 2010 per ARRA/HITECH requirements (NPRM 40872–40874) (Brodnik et al. 2012)

Changes under HITECH

Business associates face heightened obligations and penalties for noncompliance under HITECH's changes to HIPAA. These represent some of the most dramatic changes made by HITECH.

Workforce

A covered entity is responsible for ensuring that its workforce complies with HIPAA. A **workforce** includes a covered entity's paid employees. However, it also includes unpaid volunteers and trainees, and anyone who works under the covered entity's direct control whether or not the covered entity pays them (45 CFR 160.103). This also includes student interns and employees of outsourced vendors if they work routinely on the covered entity's premises (Brodnik et al. 2012). Defining an individual as a workforce member becomes important for HIPAA training purposes because covered entities and business associates are responsible for ensuring that all their workforce members are knowledgeable about HIPAA.

Section 3: What Is Covered by HIPAA

Protected Health Information (PHI)

The Privacy Rule safeguards **protected health information** (PHI) across all mediums (such as paper, electronic, imaged). To be PHI, information collected from an individual must meet a three-part test. It must be deemed "individually identifiable" by meeting the first two parts of the test:

1. It must either identify the person or provide a reasonable basis to believe the person could be identified from the information given (including demographic information).

2. It must relate to an individual's past, present, or future: physical or mental health condition; provision of healthcare; or payment for the provision of healthcare (45 CFR 160.103).

It must also then meet the third part of the three-part test to be PHI:

3. It must be held or transmitted by a covered entity or its BA in any form or medium, including electronic, paper, and oral forms (45 CFR 160.103).

Electronic vs. Paper vs. Oral Protected Health Information

If information meets the definition of PHI as explained previously, is it always protected by HIPAA and subject to HIPAA's requirements? It depends. If PHI exists in any form (paper, electronic, imaged, or oral), the HIPAA Privacy Rule applies. Therefore, improper elevator conversations involving individuals' PHI are subject to the HIPAA Privacy Rule even though they do not involve information that has been committed to paper or electronic media. The HIPAA Security Rule, however, only applies to electronic PHI. Although a covered entity or BA should protect all PHI, the distinction is important when determining the scope of the rules and whether or not violations have occurred.

Deidentified Information

The first part of the test described is important in determining whether information is PHI. It requires that information either directly identifies a person or provides a reasonable basis to believe the person could be identified from the information. If information does not meet this part of the test (even if it meets the remaining two parts), it is considered deidentified information and is not protected by HIPAA.

Deidentified information has personal characteristics removed from it. It does not identify the individual nor is there a reasonable basis to believe it could identify an individual. Because information technology is powerful, it is often possible to identify individuals by combining specific data (Brodnik et al. 2012). To ensure appropriate deidentification, HIPAA provides two options:

1. Remove 18 defined elements to ensure the patient's information is deidentified (45 CFR 164.514(b)(2)(i)).

2. Use an expert to apply generally accepted statistical and scientific principles and methods to determine the risk that the information might be used to identify an individual is minimal (45 CFR 164.514(b)(1)).

The 18 elements that must be removed for deidentification to occur are listed in figure 2.5. Identifiers that relate not only to the individual, but also to the individual's relatives, employers, and household members must be removed.

FIGURE 2.5. **Eighteen HIPAA identifiers**

1. Names

2. Geographic subdivisions smaller than a state, including street address, city, county, precinct, and zip code if that geographic unit contains fewer than 20,000 people; the initial three digits of such zip code may be changed to 000 or zip codes with the same three initial digits may be combined to form a unit of more than 20,000 people

3. All elements of dates, except the year, directly related to an individual including birth, admission, discharge, and death dates; in addition, all ages over 89 and all elements of dates (including the year) that would identify such age cannot be used, however, individuals over 89 can be aggregated into a single category of 90 or over

4. Telephone numbers

5. Fax numbers

6. E-mail addresses

7. Social Security numbers

8. Medical record numbers

9. Health plan beneficiary numbers

10. Account numbers

11. Certificate and license numbers

12. Vehicle identifiers and serial numbers, including license plate numbers

13. Device identifiers and serial numbers

14. Web Universal Resource Locators (URLs)

15. Internet Protocol (IP) address numbers

16. Biometric identifiers, including fingerprints and voice prints

17. Full face photographic images and any comparable images

18. Any other unique identifying number, characteristic, or code, except for permissible reidentification

Source: 45 CFR 164.514(b)(2)(i)

At times, a covered entity may need to reidentify deidentified PHI (that is, match it back to the individual). HIPAA permits a code to be assigned to deidentified information for reidentification. However, the code must not relate to information about the patient so that it can be translated to his or her identity. The code may not be used or disclosed for any other purpose, and it may not disclose the reidentification mechanism (Brodnik et al. 2012).

Deidentified information is often important in research studies and in operations where aggregate information can be valuable to an organization, but identification of individuals is not necessary.

Limited Data Set

A concept related to deidentified information is the limited data set. A **limited data set** is PHI that does not completely deidentify an individual, but it excludes most direct identifiers of the individual, the individual's relatives, employers, and household members (AHIMA 2012). Deidentification restrictions are lifted for ages and dates, elements of geographic subdivisions (for example, postal address information cannot be included but town or city, state, and zip code can be included) and other unique identifying information. The distinction between a limited data set and deidentified data is important because without completely deidentifying an individual HIPAA permits a limited data set to be used without a patient's authorization or opportunity to verbally agree or object for research purposes, public health, or healthcare operations as long as a data use agreement is in place to provide satisfactory assurances that the information will only be used or disclosed for the specified limited purpose. A **data use agreement** is a document that sets the parameters for permitted uses and disclosures by the recipient of the limited data set. The agreement must describe prohibitions on subsequent disclosures, provide for appropriate safeguards and reporting of inappropriate disclosures, and ensure that the recipient's agents adhere to the same parameters. The recipient must also agree not to identify the information nor contact the individuals about whom the information pertains (45 CFR 164.514(e)).

CHECK YOUR UNDERSTANDING 2.1

Instructions: Indicate whether the following statements are true or false (T or F).

1. A covered entity is training its workforce on the HIPAA Privacy Rule. It has scheduled all of its paid employees to attend training sessions. This covered entity has scheduled everyone that needs to receive training.
2. The HIPAA Security Rule applies to all types of PHI, including information disclosed verbally.
3. To be PHI, information must directly name the individual that the information is about.
4. Deidentified information receives HIPAA Privacy Rule protection.
5. Covered entities consist only of healthcare providers.

Section 4: Other Important HIPAA Concepts

In addition to understanding to whom and what HIPAA applies, as described in sections 2 and 3, there are other terms of art that explain HIPAA's applicability.

Minimum Necessary

The **minimum necessary** requirement means that covered entities and BAs (including their workforces) must limit PHI uses, disclosures, and requests to only the amount needed to accomplish the intended purpose (45 CFR 164.502(b)(1)). In other words, people should only access information if they have a business "need to know." For example, only the minimum amount of information needed to substantiate a claim for payment should be disclosed to an individual's health insurance company.

Policies and procedures should identify persons or classes of persons in a covered entity's workforce who need to access and use PHI to perform their duties. Categories of PHI appropriate for use and access by each of those persons or classes of persons should also be identified. For example, dietary department workforce members would have access to different parts of an individual's health record than intensive care unit nurses (Brodnik et al. 2012).

The minimum necessary requirement does not apply

1. To healthcare providers for treatment
2. To the individual or the individual's personal representative
3. Pursuant to the individual's authorization
4. To the Secretary of HHS for investigations, compliance review, or enforcement
5. As required by law
6. To meet other Privacy Rule compliance requirements (45 CFR 164.502(b)(2))

Individuals

HIPAA defines an **individual** as the person who is the subject of the PHI (45 CFR 160.103). *Individual* is a HIPAA term of art that is used rather than *patients, consumers,* or *clients,* which are descriptors more commonly used by healthcare providers and laypersons to identify recipients of healthcare services.

Personal Representatives

HIPAA states that a personal representative must be treated the same as the individual regarding the use and disclosure of the individual's PHI. A **personal representative** is someone who has legal authority to act on behalf of another in making healthcare decisions (45 CFR 164.502(g)). Although parents are generally the personal representatives of their minor children and have broad legal authority (including access to the minor's record), parents, guardians, or others acting *in loco parentis* (in the place of a parent) of a minor are not personal representatives if the minor has consented to his or her own treatment. Rights may also be denied to personal representatives suspected of abusing or neglecting the individual, if it is believed that granting rights could endanger the individual (Brodnik et al. 2012).

Designated Record Set

HIPAA (45 CFR 164.522, 164.524, and 164.526) allows individuals to inspect, obtain a copy of, restrict, and amend information in their designated record set, including information that exists in paper, imaged, and electronic form.

A **designated record set** (DRS) consists of records maintained by or for a covered entity including medical records; billing records; and enrollment, payment, claims adjudication, and case or medical management record systems. In each case, the records are used in whole or in part to make decisions about individuals (AHIMA 2012). A DRS includes financial information as well as information about the individual's treatment. If they are retained or used to make decisions about an individual, records should be considered to be part of the DRS even if they were not created by the covered entity or if they are **shadow records**, such as duplicate photocopied records that are maintained separately from the official health record (Brodnik et al. 2012). A covered entity must define its DRS and identify where it is located, which can be in one or more places. This process is important regardless of whether the health record is paper, imaged, electronic or a **hybrid health record** (that is, a combination of paper and electronic).

The DRS distinction is important because information that is not part of a DRS is not subject to HIPAA, such as an individual's right of access. For example, telephone messages, surgery schedules, and appointment logs are not part of the DRS because they are not used to make healthcare or payment decisions about an individual (Brodnik et al. 2012). Figure 2.6 provides types of documents that would not be part of the designated record set.

FIGURE 2.6.	Documents not included in the designated record set
Outside the Designated Record Set	**Examples**
Health information generated, collected, or maintained for purposes that do not include decision making about the individual	• Data collected and maintained for research • Data collected and maintained for peer review purposes • Data collected and maintained for performance improvement purposes • Appointment and surgery schedules • Birth and death registers • Surgery registers • Diagnostic or operative indexes • Duplicate copies of information that can also be located in the individual's medical or billing record
Psychotherapy notes	The notes of a mental health professional about counseling sessions that are maintained separate and apart from the regular health record
Information compiled in reasonable anticipation of or for use in a civil, criminal, or administrative action or proceeding	Notes taken by a covered entity during a meeting with the covered entity's attorney about a pending lawsuit

FIGURE 2.6.	(Continued)
Outside the Designated Record Set	**Examples**
Clinical Laboratory Improvement Amendments CLIA	• Requisitions for laboratory tests • Duplicate lab results when the originals are filed in the individual's paper chart
Employer records	• Pre-employment physicals maintained in human resource files • The results of HIV tests maintained by the infectious disease control nurse on employees who have suffered needle stick injuries on the job
Business associate records that meet the definition of designated record set but that merely duplicate information maintained by the covered entity	Transcribed operative reports that have been transmitted to the covered entity
Education records	Records generated and maintained by teachers and teachers' aides employed by a school district or patients in acute care hospitals, institutions for the developmentally disabled, and rehabilitation care centers
Source (raw) data interpreted or summarized in the individual's medical or health record	• Pathology slides • Diagnostic films • Electrocardiogram tracings from which interpretations are derived
Versions	Management of multiple revisions of the same document. By versioning, each iteration of a document is tracked.
Metadata	Data that provides a detailed description about other data. "Information about a particular data set or document that describes how, when, and by whom it was collected, created, accessed, or modified and how it is formatted."
Audits	Results of reviews to identify variations from established baselines or used to track an individual's activity in an electronic system (for example, view, print, edit).
Pending reports	Reports that have been initiated by a member of the healthcare team but are not yet authenticated and may not be available for viewing by staff until completed. An EHR system will keep these documents in a pending or incomplete status.

Source: AHIMA 2011

Business associates often have records that meet the DRS definition. If they do, then the records are part of the covered entity's DRS. If PHI is not used to make decisions about individuals (for example, quality improvement activities), it is not part of the DRS even though it is in the custody of a covered entity (Brodnik et al. 2012).

Distinguishing the Legal Health Record

The DRS is different than the **legal health record** (LHR). The LHR is an organization's official business record and consists of documents and data elements that may be disclosed in response to legally permissible requests for patient information (AHIMA 2012). It is generally limited to information related to treatment of a patient. Organizations must determine their own definition of the LHR and what suits their needs. As a result, its content will vary from one covered entity to the next. However, as opposed to the broader DRS that includes all PHI, the LHR does not include billing and claims payment records. The LHR may consist of paper, imaged or electronic media, or a combination of these formats. Figure 2.7 provides a comparison between the DRS and the legal health record.

There are certain types of data not included in the designated record set or the legal health record. They include data used for administrative, regulatory, financial, and operational purposes. Examples include electronic health record audit trails that trace access, changes and additions to health records; correspondence requesting health records; and databases that contain patient information. Derived data—aggregated or summarized data that does not identify the patient—includes statistical reports, accreditation reports, and anonymous patient data that has been compiled for research (AHIMA 2011).

Disclosure, Use, and Request

HIPAA addresses three ways that PHI is handled: disclosure, use, and request. **Disclosure** is the dissemination of PHI from a covered entity or BA. **Use** is the handling of PHI that is internal to a covered entity or BA. Such functions include utilization, examination, and analysis (AHIMA 2012). Covered entities and BAs must also comply with HIPAA when they **request** or ask for access to PHI. HIPAA emphasizes disclosure and use.

Treatment, Payment, and Healthcare Operations

Treatment, payment, and healthcare operations (TPO) are, collectively, a covered entity's functions necessary to successfully conduct business (AHIMA 2012). Some of HIPAA's requirements are relaxed or removed where an individual's PHI is needed to carry out TPO. Otherwise, HIPAA would impose too great of restrictions on carrying out these essential functions. For example, HIPAA's authorization requirement is not applicable to disclosures of PHI from one physician to another if the disclosure is for treatment purposes.

Treatment is providing, coordinating, or managing healthcare services by healthcare providers. It also includes healthcare provider consultations and referrals. For example, PHI that provides background information about an individual may be sent from the individual's family physician to a cardiologist to facilitate a cardiac consultation for the individual.

The definition of **payment** is broad. It includes a health plan's activities to obtain premiums or a healthcare provider's activities to obtain reimbursement for care or services provided. Other activities included in the payment definition are billing, claims management, claims collection, review of the medical necessity of care, and utilization review. HIPAA's **healthcare operations** definition is also broad. It includes quality improvement, case management, review of healthcare professionals' qualifications, insurance contracting, legal and auditing functions, and functions such as customer service (Brodnik et al. 2012).

FIGURE 2.7.	Comparison of designated record set (DRS) and legal health record (LHR)

This side-by-side comparison of the designated record set and the legal health record demonstrates the differences between the two sets of information, as well as their purposes.

	Designated Record Set	Legal Health Record
Definition	A group of records maintained by or for a covered entity that is the medical and billing records about individuals; enrollment, payment, claims adjudication, and case or medical management record systems maintained by or for a health plan; information used in whole or in part by or for the HIPAA covered entity to make decisions about individuals.	The business record generated at or for a healthcare organization. It is the record that would be released upon receipt of a request. The legal health record is the officially declared record of healthcare services provided to an individual delivered by a provider.
Purpose	Used to clarify the access and amendment standards in the HIPAA Privacy Rule, which provide that individuals generally have the right to inspect and obtain a copy of protected health information in the designated record set.	The official business record of healthcare services delivered by the entity for regulatory and disclosure purposes.
Content	Defined in organizational policy and required by the HIPAA Privacy Rule. The content of the designated record set includes medical and billing records of covered providers; enrollment, payment, claims, and case information of a health plan; and information used in whole or in part by or for the covered entity to make decisions about individuals.	Defined in organizational policy and can include individually identifiable data in any medium collected and directly used in documenting healthcare services or health status. It excludes administrative, derived, and aggregate data.
Uses	Supports individual HIPAA right of access and amendment.	Provides a record of health status as well as documentation of care for reimbursement, quality management, research, and public health purposes; facilitates business decision making and education of healthcare practitioners as well as the legal needs of the healthcare organization.

Source: AHIMA 2011

Of the range of TPO activities, only treatment is exempt from the minimum necessary requirement discussed previously. PHI used or disclosed for payment and operations must be limited to the minimum necessary.

Health Information in Personnel and Educational Records

Covered entities and BAs are subject to HIPAA, but HIPAA does not apply to all information they hold or come into contact with (recall that it only protects PHI). For example, HIPAA excludes a covered entity's employment records that it holds as an employer (45 CFR 160.103). Therefore, employee physical examination reports in personnel files are not protected by HIPAA. Educational records covered by the Federal Educational Records Privacy Act (FERPA) (20 USC 1232(g)) are also not protected by HIPAA because they are not defined as PHI (Brodnik et al. 2012).

Organization Types

Covered entity is a term of art under HIPAA and encompasses healthcare providers, health plans, and healthcare clearinghouses. However, these categories are not mutually exclusive or all-inclusive. One aspect of an organization may function as a covered entity while another aspect of that same business does not. Further, an organization may function as more than one type of covered entity.

A **hybrid entity** performs both covered and noncovered functions under HIPAA (45 CFR 164.103). One example of a hybrid entity is a university. The aspect of that organization that educates students and maintains student educational records is not covered by HIPAA; however, the same university may operate a hospital or medical center. That aspect of the business (healthcare provider) is covered by HIPAA.

An **affiliated covered entity** refers to legally separate covered entities affiliated by common ownership or control (45 CFR 164.105). For purposes of HIPAA, the separate entities may refer to themselves as a single covered entity. For example, a hospital and its associated physician practices may be an affiliated covered entity.

An **organized healthcare arrangement** consists of two or more covered entities that share an individual's PHI as a way to manage and benefit their common enterprise (45 CFR 164.103). They are recognized by the public as a single entity. For example, a large medical center may have an acute care facility and a behavioral health facility. These two facilities may be part of one organized healthcare arrangement, enabling them to share individual information with each other.

It is possible for covered entities to perform multiple functions covered by HIPAA (45 CFR 164.504(g)). Each covered function must be operated separately so that individual's PHI is not disclosed to a function not involved with the individual. An example is a medical facility that also operates as a self-insured health plan. An employee of the facility may be a patient at the facility, but not an enrollee of the health plan. The individual's PHI may only be used by the medical facility in its role as a healthcare provider. The information cannot be shared with the health plan (Brodnik et al. 2012).

CHECK YOUR UNDERSTANDING 2.2

Instructions: Indicate whether the following statements are true or false (T or F).

1. Under HIPAA, a personal representative must be treated the same as the individual regarding the use and disclosure of the individual's PHI.
2. By definition, a designated record set includes billing records.
3. A hospital employee's pre-employment physical examination is in his personnel file in Human Resources; this report is protected by HIPAA.
4. A university with a medical center is a hybrid entity under HIPAA.
5. Some of the Privacy Rule's requirements are relaxed or removed where an individual's PHI is needed to carry out TPO.

REAL-WORLD CASE

What, exactly, is deidentified information? This chapter and the accompanying figure 2.5 seem to provide a fairly clear answer. However, a tragic case demonstrates that the answer is not always straightforward. An 18-year-old male high school student lived in a community of approximately 40,000 people and was a member of the high school basketball team. He died after the car in which he was a passenger struck a tree in a high-speed crash. The young man's health records were disclosed without authorization by the provider and later used as a case study in a high school class discussion about driving safety. Although his name and other obvious identifiers such as date of birth and Social Security number were not used, because the nature of his injuries was unique it was apparent to those who knew him and those who were aware of the accident that the records being used were those of the student.

It was concluded that no state law was violated, although a state law was subsequently passed requiring that healthcare providers have policies in place to limit "the use and disclosure of medical records, images, videos, or pictures intended to be used for medical educational purposes …" and it further requires protocols for written authorizations (Colby Stansberry Act 2010). Apparently no HIPAA complaint was filed either. However, this case brings into focus the 18th (and final) identifier: Any other unique identifying number, characteristic, or code, except for permissible reidentification. Although this case may not represent the norm with respect to deidentification, it highlights—through a tragic set of circumstances—that removal of all clearly stated identifiers may not deidentify PHI and that all 18 identifiers set forth in HIPAA, including the final identifier, must be carefully considered.

SUMMARY

HIPAA is a broad statute governing many areas in addition to privacy and security. From this statute, however, come the HIPAA Privacy and Security Rules. These rules drive the protection of patient information. From this chapter, the reader should understand key concepts that serve as underpinnings to HIPAA's protection of patient information. This understanding should include the knowledge that while HIPAA casts a wide net, it is not all-encompassing. This chapter explained *to whom* and *to what* HIPAA applies, as well as describing terms of art the reader will need to know in order to understand any further HIPAA implications.

REFERENCES

American Health Information Management Association. 2011. Fundamentals of the legal health record and designated record set. *Journal of AHIMA* 82(2): 44–49.

American Health Information Management Association. 2012. *Pocket Glossary for Health Information Management and Technology*, 3rd ed. Chicago: AHIMA.

Brodnik, M., L. Rinehart-Thompson, and R. Reynolds. 2012. *Fundamentals of Law for Health Informatics and Information Management*, 2nd ed. Chicago: AHIMA.

Cassidy, B. 2000. HIPAA on the job: Update on business partner/associate agreements. *Journal of AHIMA* 71(10):16A–16D.

Colby Stansberry Act: Tennessee Code Annotated 63-2-101(b)(3). 2010.

Walsh, T. 2011. AHIMA Practice Brief: Security risk analysis and management: An overview (updated). *Journal of AHIMA* http://library.ahima.org/xpedio/groups/public/documents/ahima/bok1_048622 .hcsp?dDocName=bok1_048622.

20 USC §1232(g): Federal Educational Records Privacy Act (FERPA). 1974.

45 CFR 160: General Administrative Requirements. 2006.

45 CFR 160.103: Definitions. 2006.

45 CFR 160.103(1): Business associate. 2006.

45 CFR 164: Security and Privacy. 2006.

45 CFR 164.103: Definitions. 2006.

45 CFR 164.105: Organizational requirements. 2006.

45 CFR 164.502(b)(1): Uses and disclosures of protected health information: general rules. Standard: minimum necessary. Minimum necessary applies. 2006.

45 CFR 164.502(b)(2): Uses and disclosures of protected health information: general rules. Standard: minimum necessary. Minimum necessary does not apply. 2006.

45 CFR 164.502(g): Uses and disclosures of protected health information: general rules. Standard: personal representatives. 2006.

45 CFR 164.306(a): Security standards: General rules. General requirements. 2006.

45 CFR 164.504(g): Uses and disclosures: organizational requirements. Standard: requirements for a covered entity with multiple covered functions. 2006.

45 CFR 164.514(b)(1)): Other requirements relating to uses and disclosures of protected health information. Implementation specifications: requirements for de-identification of protected health information. 2006.

45 CFR 164.514(b)(2)(i): Other requirements relating to uses and disclosures of protected health information. Implementation specifications: requirements for de-identification of protected health information. 2006.

45 CFR 164.514(e): Other requirements relating to uses and disclosures of protected health information. Standard: limited data set. 2006.

45 CFR 164.522: Rights to request privacy protection for protected health information. 2006.

45 CFR 164.524: Access of individuals to protected health information. 2006.

45 CFR 164.526: Amendment of protected health information. 2006.

CHAPTER **3**

HIPAA Privacy Rule Concepts

Learning Objectives

- Compare the purposes and elements of the Notice of Privacy Practices, consent, and authorization

- Analyze situations that do and do not require patient authorization per HIPAA

- Discuss the concept of preemption and explain when it would apply

- Discuss examples of each of the individual rights granted by HIPAA

- Explain HIPAA's requirements on the use of protected health information for marketing and fundraising purposes

- Explain HIPAA's parameters on the use of protected health information for research

- Summarize the administrative requirements imposed by HIPAA

KEY TERMS

Access

Accounting of disclosures

Altered authorization

Amendment

Authorization

Clinical Laboratory Improvements
  Amendments (CLIA) of 1988

Compound authorizations

Conditioned authorizations

Confidential communications

Consent

Facility directory

Fundraising

Health Insurance Portability and
  Accountability Act (HIPAA) of 1996

HIPAA Privacy Rule

HIPAA Security Rule

Incidental uses and disclosures

Institutional Review Board (IRB)

Limited data set

Marketing

Mitigation

Notice of Privacy Practices (NPP)

Office for Civil Rights (OCR)

Preemption

Privacy board

Privacy officer

Psychotherapy notes

Restriction request

Retaliation and waiver

Stand-alone authorizations

Treatment, payment, and healthcare
  operations (TPO)

Unconditioned authorizations

United States Department of Health and
  Human Services (HHS)

Waived authorization

Workforce

INTRODUCTION

The **Health Insurance Portability and Accountability Act (HIPAA)** of 1996 Privacy and Security Rules are key federal regulations governing the privacy and security of health information. The **HIPAA Privacy Rule** places a greater emphasis on policies and procedures. The **HIPAA Security Rule**, which applies only to electronic protected health information (PHI), emphasizes technology. They reside in 45 CFR Parts 160 and 164. This chapter will discuss the Privacy Rule (which will be referred to as HIPAA throughout the chapter). The Security Rule will be detailed in chapter 4.

HIPAA has two goals. The first goal is to provide an individual with greater rights regarding his or her health information. The second goal is to provide greater privacy protections for one's health information, including limited access by others. This chapter will detail requirements that carry out these two goals.

Section 1: Key Documents

HIPAA addresses three primary documents that inform patients and give them a measure of control over their PHI. Two of these documents, the Notice of Privacy Practices and the authorization, are required. The third, consent, is optional. Figure 3.1 outlines differences among these three key documents.

FIGURE 3.1.	Notice of Privacy Practices, consent, and authorization		
	Notice of Privacy Practices	**Consent**	**Authorization**
Required?	Required by HIPAA	Optional	Required by HIPAA
Requirements re: TPO	Must explain TPO uses and disclosures, along with other types of uses and disclosures	Obtains patient permission to use or disclose PHI for TPO purposes only	Is used to obtain for a number of types of uses and disclosures, although is not required for TPO uses and disclosures
PHI that this document addresses	Provides prospective and general information about how PHI might be used or disclosed in the future (and includes information that may not have been created yet)	Provides prospective and general information about how PHI might be used or disclosed in the future for TPO purposes (and includes information that may not have been created yet)	Obtains patient permission to use or disclose specific information that generally has already been created and for which there is a specific need
Required for treatment?	May not refuse to treat an individual because he or she declines to sign this form	May condition treatment on individual signing this form	May not refuse to treat an individual because he or she declines to sign this form
Time limit on document validity	No time limit on validity of the document	No time limit on validity of the document	Time limit on validity of document (specified by an expiration date or event)

Source: Brodnik et al. 2012

Notice of Privacy Practices

It is important for individuals to have some control over—or at least knowledge of—uses and disclosures of their health information. Educating individuals about how their PHI is used or disclosed is one of the main purposes of the Notice of Privacy Practices.

An individual generally has the right to a **Notice of Privacy Practices (NPP)** that is written in plain language and explains how a covered entity will use his or her PHI (45 CFR 164.520). The NPP also explains an individual's rights and the covered entity's legal duties regarding PHI. An individual must be given the NPP at his or her first contact with the covered entity (for example, the first visit to a physician's office or first admission to a hospital). Parents of minor children must be given an NPP. After an individual's first encounter, unless there are material changes, the NPP does not have to be given to an individual again. However, it must be made available upon request. Figure 3.2 provides a sample NPP.

FIGURE 3.2.	Sample Notice of Privacy Practices

THIS NOTICE DESCRIBES HOW INFORMATION ABOUT YOU MAY BE USED AND DISCLOSED AND HOW YOU CAN GET ACCESS TO THIS INFORMATION. PLEASE REVIEW IT CAREFULLY.

Understanding Your Health Record/Information

Each time you visit a hospital, physician, or other healthcare provider, a record of your visit is made. Typically, this record contains your symptoms, examination and test results, diagnoses, treatment, and a plan for future care or treatment. This information, often referred to as your "health record" or "medical record," serves as a:

- Basis for planning your care and treatment
- Means of communication among the many health professionals who contribute to your care
- Legal document describing the care you received
- Means by which you or a third-party payer can verify that services billed actually were provided
- Tool in educating health professionals
- Source of data for medical research
- Source of information for public health officials charged with improving the health of the nation
- Source of data for facility planning and marketing
- Tool with which we can assess and continually work to improve the care we render and the outcomes we achieve

Understanding what is in your record and how your health information is used helps you to:

- Ensure its accuracy
- Better understand who, what, when, where, and why others may access your health information
- Make more informed decisions when authorizing disclosure to others

FIGURE 3.2. | **(Continued)**

Your Health Information Rights

Although your health record is the physical property of the healthcare practitioner or facility that compiled it, the information belongs to you. You have the right to:

- Request a restriction on certain uses and disclosures of your information as provided by 45 CFR 164.522. The covered entity is not required to agree to a requested restriction, except in case of a disclosure restricted under 164.522

- Obtain a paper copy of the notice of information practices upon request

- Inspect and copy your health record as provided for in 45 CFR 164.524

- Amend your health record as provided in 45 CFR 164.526

- Obtain an accounting of disclosures of your health information as provided in 45 CFR 164.528

- Request communications of your health information by alternative means or at alternative locations

- Revoke your authorization to use or disclose health information except to the extent that action has already been taken

Our Responsibilities

This organization is required to:

- Maintain the privacy of your health information

- Provide you with a notice as to our legal duties and privacy practices with respect to information we collect and maintain about you

- Abide by the terms of this notice

- Notify you if we are unable to agree to a requested restriction

- Accommodate reasonable requests you may have to communicate health information by alternative means or at alternative locations

The covered entity is required by law to maintain the privacy of protected health information, to provide individuals with notice of its legal duties and privacy practices with respect to protected health information, and to notify affected individuals following a breach of unsecured protected health information.

We reserve the right to change our practices and to make the new provisions effective for all protected health information we maintain. Should our information practices change, we will mail a revised notice to the address you have supplied us.

We will not use or disclose your health information without your authorization, except as described in this notice.

For More Information or to Report a Problem

If you have questions and would like additional information, you may contact the Director of Health Information Management at (444) 111–1111.

If you believe your privacy rights have been violated, you can file a complaint with the Director of Health Information Management or with the Secretary of Health and Human Services. There will be no retaliation for filing a complaint.

(Continued on next page)

FIGURE 3.2. **(Continued)**

Examples of Disclosures for Treatment, Payment, and Health Operations

We will use your health information for treatment. For example: Information obtained by a nurse, physician, or other member of your healthcare team will be recorded in your record and used to determine the course of treatment that should work best for you. Your physician will document in your record his or her expectations of the members of your healthcare team. Members of your healthcare team will then record the actions they took and their observations. In that way, the physician will know how you are responding to treatment. We will also provide your physician or a subsequent healthcare provider with copies of various reports that should assist him or her in treating you once you are discharged from this hospital.

We will use your health information for payment. For example: A bill may be sent to you or a third-party payer. The information on or accompanying the bill may include information that identifies you, as well as your diagnosis, procedures, and supplies used.

We will use your health information for regular health operations. For example: Members of the medical staff, the risk or quality improvement manager, or members of the quality improvement team may use information in your health record to assess the care and outcomes in your case and others like it. This information will then be used in an effort to continue improving the quality and effectiveness of the healthcare and service we provide.

Other Uses or Disclosures

Business associates: Some services in our organization are provided through contacts with business associates. Examples include physician services in the emergency department and radiology, certain laboratory tests, and a copy service we use when making copies of your health record. When these services are contracted, we may disclose your health information to our business associates so that they can perform the job we have asked them to do and bill you or your third-party payer for services rendered. So that your health information is protected, however, we require the business associate to safeguard your information appropriately.

Directory: Unless you notify us that you object, we will use your name, location in the facility, general condition, and religious affiliation for directory purposes. This information may be provided to members of the clergy and, except for religious affiliation, to other people who ask for you by name.

Notification: We may use or disclose information to notify or assist in notifying a family member, personal representative, or another person responsible for your care, location, and general condition.

Communication with family: Health professionals, using their best judgment, may disclose to a family member, other relative, close personal friend, or any other person you identify, health information relevant to that person's involvement in your care or payment related to your care.

Research: We may disclose information to researchers when their research has been approved by an institutional review board that has reviewed the research proposal and established protocols to ensure the privacy of your health information.

FIGURE 3.2. (Continued)

Funeral directors: We may disclose to funeral directors health information consistent with applicable law so they can carry out their duties.

Organ procurement organizations: Consistent with applicable law, for the purpose of tissue donation and transplant, we may disclose health information to organ procurement organizations or other entities engaged in the procurement, banking, or transplantation of organs.

Marketing: We may contact you to provide appointment reminders or information about treatment alternatives or other health-related benefits and services that may be of interest to you.

Fundraising: We may contact you as part of a fundraising effort and you have a right to opt out of receiving such communications.

Food and Drug Administration (FDA): We may disclose to the FDA health information relative to adverse events with respect to food, supplements, product and product defects, or postmarketing surveillance information to enable product recalls, repairs, or replacement.

Workers' compensation: We may disclose health information to the extent authorized by and to the extent necessary to comply with laws relating to workers' compensation or other similar programs established by law.

Public health: As required by law, we may disclose your health information to public health or legal authorities charged with preventing or controlling disease, injury, or disability.

Correctional institution: Should you be an inmate of a correctional institution, we may disclose to the institution or agents thereof health information necessary for your health and the health and safety of other individuals.

Law enforcement: We may disclose health information for law enforcement purposes as required by law or in response to a valid subpoena.

Federal law makes provisions for your health information to be released to an appropriate health oversight agency, public health authority, or attorney, provided that a workforce member or business associate believes in good faith that we have engaged in unlawful conduct or have otherwise violated professional or clinical standards and are potentially endangering one or more patients, workers, or the public.

My signature below indicates that I have been provided with a copy of the notice of privacy practices.	
_____	_____
Signature of Patient or Legal Representative	Date
If signed by legal representative, relationship to patient _____	
Effective Date: _____	
Distribution: Original to provider, copy to patient	

Source: AHIMA 2011b

Not all first service encounters are face-to-face. If a service is first provided by telephone (for example, a telephone consultation), the NPP must be promptly mailed after the telephone encounter. If services are first provided electronically (for example, electronic prescribing), the NPP must be delivered automatically and simultaneously. The NPP must be available at the site where the individual is treated and must be posted in a prominent place where the individual can reasonably be expected to read it. A covered entity's website must prominently post the NPP. If an individual's first encounter with a covered entity is in an emergency situation, the covered entity must provide the NPP to the individual as soon as possible after the emergency.

If an individual requests a copy of the NPP, even if it is not the first service encounter, it must be provided. Good-faith attempts must be made to obtain written acknowledgment from the individual that he or she received the notice. Failure to obtain acknowledgment must be documented, whether due to patient refusal or noncompliance or failure by the covered entity (45 CFR 164.520(c)(2)).

Consent

HIPAA does not require healthcare providers to obtain the individual's **consent** to use or disclose PHI for **treatment, payment, and healthcare operations (TPO)** (45 CFR 164.506(b)). However, some providers choose to obtain it when healthcare services are provided. When HIPAA requires an authorization, consent cannot serve as a substitute. Because it has no expiration date, consent is generally indefinite unless the individual specifically revokes it.

Obtaining consent may be difficult or impossible (for example, in an emergency situation). If it is a provider's policy to obtain consent but it cannot be obtained prior to treatment, the provider should document the attempt and the reason it was unable to do so. The provider should then obtain consent as soon as possible (for example, after emergency treatment has been given).

Authorization

HIPAA specifies when an individual's written **authorization** is required for disclosure of PHI. Under HIPAA, a valid authorization must be written in plain language. Other requirements include identifying the name of the patient whose PHI is being disclosed; identifying the type of information to be disclosed and to whom the disclosure may be made; and providing for the signature of the patient or patient's authorized legal representative. An authorization must contain at least the elements listed in figure 3.3. An authorization is defective if any of the occurrences listed in figure 3.4 take place. Defects include use of the authorization despite expiration dates that have passed; use of the authorization although it is known that material information is false; and the lack of any of the required elements listed in figure 3.3. Figure 3.5 displays a sample authorization form. Required elements for a valid authorization are included on this form. An individual may revoke an authorization at any time if it is done in writing. A revocation does not apply if the covered entity has already acted on the authorization.

FIGURE 3.3.	Elements required by the Privacy Rule for a valid authorization

#	**Section 1: Requirements for Authorization to Disclose Patient Health Information or Records (45 CFR §164.508(c) — HIPAA)**
1	Authorization is written in plain language.
2	Authorization identifies the name of the patient whose PHI is being disclosed.
3	Authorization identifies the type of information to be disclosed.
4	Authorization identifies the names or classes of persons or types of healthcare providers authorized to make the disclosure.
5	Authorization identifies the names or classes of persons or types of healthcare providers authorized to whom the organization may make the disclosure.
6	Authorization identifies the purpose of the disclosure.
7	Authorization contains the signature of the patient or patient's authorized legal representative.
8	If signed by an authorized legal representative, the authorization identifies the relationship of that person to the patient.
9	Authorization includes the date on which the authorization is signed.
10	Authorization identifies the time period for which the authorization is effective and expiration date or event.
11	Authorization contains a statement informing the individual regarding the right to revoke the authorization in writing and a description how to do so.
12	Authorization contains a statement informing the individual about the organization's ability or inability to condition treatment, payment, enrollment, or eligibility for benefits.
13	Authorization contains a statement informing the individual about the potential for information to be redisclosed and no longer protected by the federal privacy rule.
14	Authorization contains a statement that if an organization is seeking the authorization, a copy must be provided to the individual signing the authorization.
15	Authorization contains a statement that the individual may inspect or copy the health information disclosed.
16	Authorization includes a statement regarding assessment of reasonable fees for copy services.

(Continued on next page)

FIGURE 3.3. (Continued)

Section 2: Additional Requirements for Authorization to Disclose Sensitive or Restricted Health Information (Refer to Applicable Federal and State Laws for Categories Below)

Mental health or behavioral health patient health information or records

Alcohol or other drug abuse patient health information or records

Developmental disability patient health information or records

HIV test results or patient health information or records

Other: sexual abuse, child abuse, elder abuse, and the like

The Department of Health and Human Services offered the following guidance about authorizations:

"The Privacy Rule requires that an Authorization contain either an expiration date or an expiration event that relates to the individual or the purpose of the use or disclosure. For example, an Authorization may expire 'one year from the date the Authorization is signed,' 'upon the minor's age of majority,' or 'upon termination of enrollment in the health plan'" (HHS 2003).

"An Authorization remains valid until its expiration date or event, unless effectively revoked in writing by the individual before that date or event" (HHS 2003).

Source: AHIMA 2012(a)

FIGURE 3.4. Defective authorizations

An authorization is defective if any of the following occurs:

- The expiration date has passed or the covered entity knows the expiration event has occurred.
- The authorization has not been filled out completely for a required element or lacks a required element.
- The covered entity knows the authorization has been revoked.
- The authorization violates the compound authorization requirements, if applicable. (A compound authorization combines an individual's authorization for the disclosure of health information with informed consent for the performance of medical treatment.)
- The covered entity knows that material information in the authorization is false.
- Completion of an authorization is required for an individual to be eligible for treatment, payment, or enrollment in a health plan, or to be eligible for benefits on an authorization (with certain exceptions to this rule delineated in 45 CFR 164.508(b)(4)).

Source: 45 CFR 164.508(b)(2)

HIPAA specifically addresses **psychotherapy notes**, which are behavioral health notes recorded by a mental health professional who documents or analyzes contents and impressions of conversations that are part of private counseling sessions. Psychotherapy notes are separated from the rest of an individual's health record and do not contain information such as start and stop times, prescriptions and monitoring, treatment modalities and frequencies, or test results. Further, they do not summarize the individual's symptoms, diagnosis, prognosis, treatment plan, functional status, or progress to date (45 CFR 164.501). Authorizations are always required for the use or disclosure of psychotherapy notes except to carry out TPO for the purposes of rendering treatment by the originator of the notes, conducting counseling training, or defending a legal action brought by the individual (45 CFR 164.508(a)(2)).

FIGURE 3.5.	Sample authorization to disclose health information

Patient Last Name: _____ Patient First Name: _____

Address: _____

Phone Number: _____ Date of Birth: _____

Health Record Number: _____

1. I authorize the disclosure of the above named individual's health information as described below. Please specify requested dates of service:

2. The following individual(s) or organization(s) are authorized to make the disclosure:

   Name: _____

   Address: _____

3. The type of information to be disclosed is as follows (check the appropriate boxes and include other information where indicated)

   - problem list
   - medication list
   - list of allergies
   - immunization records
   - most recent history
   - most recent discharge summary
   - laboratory test results (please describe the dates or types of test results you would like disclosed):
   - x-ray or imaging report(s) (please specify the date and type of each report requested):

     _____

   - x-ray or imaging film(s) (please specify the date and type of each film requested):

     _____

(Continued on next page)

FIGURE 3.5. **(Continued)**

- consultation reports from (please supply doctors' names):

  _____

- entire record
- other (please describe):

  _____

4. I understand that the information in my health record may include information relating to sexually transmitted disease, acquired immunodeficiency syndrome (AIDS), or human immunodeficiency virus (HIV). It may also include information about behavioral or mental health services and treatment for alcohol and drug abuse.

5. The information identified above may be disclosed to the following individuals or organization(s):
   Name: _____
   Address: _____
   Name: _____
   Address: _____

6. This information for which I am authorizing disclosure will be used for the following purpose:
   - my personal records
   - sharing with other healthcare providers as needed
   - other (please describe):

   _____

7. I understand that I have a right to revoke this authorization at any time. I understand that if I revoke this authorization, I must do so in writing and present my written revocation to the health information management department. I understand that the revocation will not apply to information that has already been released in response to this authorization. I understand that the revocation will not apply to my insurance company when the law provides my insurer with the right to contest a claim under my policy.

8. This authorization will expire (insert date or event):

   _____

   If I fail to specify an expiration date or event, this authorization will expire six months from the date on which it was signed.

9. I understand that once the above information is disclosed, it may be redisclosed by the recipient and the information may not be protected by federal privacy laws or regulations.

10. I understand authorizing the disclosure of the information identified above is voluntary. I need not sign this form to ensure healthcare treatment.

FIGURE 3.5.	Sample authorization to disclose health information

Signature of patient or legal representative: _____

Date: _____

If signed by legal representative, relationship to patient: _____

Signature of witness: _____

Date: _____

Distribution of copies: Original to provider; copy to patient; copy to accompany disclosure

Note: The types of documents listed on the authorization form may need to be modified for the particular healthcare setting. Authorizations for marketing need to disclose whether remuneration was received by the covered entity.

Source: AHIMA 2012(b)

Section 2: Use and Disclosure When Authorization Is Not Required

The general rule under HIPAA regarding authorizations is that an individual's written authorization is required for the use or disclosure of his or her PHI unless the situation is an exception where written authorization is not required.

Stated another way, unless HIPAA specifically mentions circumstances where written authorization is not required for a use or disclosure, it is required. Note that a verbal agreement to use or disclose an individual's PHI is not the same as an authorization, which must be in writing. Figure 3.6 outlines when an authorization is and is not required. Covered entities must consider HIPAA's authorization requirements in conjunction with state laws governing authorization for use and disclosure.

Use and Disclosure Required without Authorization

There are only two situations where HIPAA *requires* use or disclosure of PHI without the individual's authorization. These are when the individual (or the individual's personal representative) requests access to PHI or an accounting of disclosures of the PHI, and when the **United States Department of Health and Human Services (HHS)** is conducting an investigation, review, or enforcement action.

Use and Disclosure Permitted without Authorization

There are many situations where HIPAA *permits* a covered entity to use or disclose PHI without an individual's authorization (45 CFR 164.510; 45 CFR 164.512), as outlined in figure 3.6. This means that use or disclosure without authorization will not result in a HIPAA violation. There may be stricter state laws that do not allow the use or disclosure without authorization. Also, a covered entity's policy may require patient authorization even if HIPAA permits use or disclosure without it. For example, a hospital is not required by HIPAA to obtain a patient's authorization before sending hospital records to a physician

FIGURE 3.6. Authorization requirements for use and disclosure of PHI

I. Patient Authorization Required:

All situations except those listed in Part II

II. Patient Authorization Not Required:

A. When use or disclosure is required, even without patient authorization

- When the individual or the individual's personal representative requests access or accountings of disclosures (with exceptions)
- Dept. of HHS investigation, review, or enforcement action

B. When use or disclosure is permitted, even without patient authorization

- Patient has opportunity to informally agree or object
  - o facility directory
  - o notification of relatives and friends
- Patient does not have opportunity to agree or object
  - o Public interest and benefit (12 types)

    1. As required by law

    2. For public health activities

    3. To disclose PHI regarding victims of abuse, neglect, or domestic violence

    4. For health over sight activities

    5. For judicial and administrative proceedings

    6. For law enforcement purpose (six specific situations)

    7. Regarding decedents

    8. For cadaveric organ, eye, or tissue donation

    9. For research, with limitations

    10. To prevent or lessen serious threat to health or safety

    11. For essential government function

    12. For workers' compensation
  - o TPO
  - o To the individual/patient
  - o Incidental uses and disclosures
  - o Limited data sets

Source: Brodnik et al. 2012

for follow-up (that is, treatment purposes). However, its policy may require that patient authorization be obtained anyway.

Opportunity to Agree or Object

There are two situations where HIPAA does not require authorization, but the patient must be informed in advance and be given the opportunity to informally (that is, verbally) agree, object, or restrict the use or disclosure (45 CFR 164.510). The first situation is inclusion in a **facility directory** of patients currently being treated. If an individual agrees, HIPAA permits the facility to share the following with persons who ask for the individual by name: name, location in the facility, condition described in general terms. Clergy members of an individual's religious affiliation may receive a list of all patients of that affiliation. The individual must be given the opportunity to restrict or prohibit some or all of the uses or disclosures.

In emergencies, if it is impractical or impossible to inform the patient and obtain agreement, a patient can temporarily be listed in the facility directory if it is consistent with the prior expressed preference of the patient or is determined to be in the patient's best interest. As soon as possible after the emergency, the patient must be informed and given the opportunity to agree or object to inclusion in the facility directory.

The second situation where HIPAA does not require authorization, but the patient must be informed in advance and be given the opportunity to informally (that is, verbally) agree or object, is disclosure of relevant PHI to a family member, relative, or close friend who is involved in the individual's care or payment. If the individual agrees, this allows, for example, those acting on behalf of the individual to accomplish things such as picking up prescriptions. If the individual is not present or is unable to agree or object, a covered entity may use its professional judgment to decide if disclosure is in the individual's best interest. Only relevant information may be disclosed (45 CFR 164.510(b)), but this also allows a covered entity to notify a family member or other person who is responsible for the individual's care.

There are two situations in which the covered entity may disclose relevant PHI. The first is for the purpose of coordinating with designated entities for disaster relief. The covered entity may use professional judgment to determine what information may be used and disclosed for disaster relief. The second, a covered entity may disclose PHI on a deceased individual to a family member or other person who is involved with the individual's care or payment for healthcare prior to the individual's death, provided that this is consistent with the deceased individual's preferences, that is to know the covered entity.

Opportunity to Agree or Object Not Required

There are 16 circumstances where HIPAA permits PHI to be used or disclosed without either the individual's written authorization or an opportunity to verbally agree, object, or restrict. The first 12 circumstances (informally referred to as public interest and benefit activities) have been identified as serving national priorities (45 CFR 164.512). However, if the use or disclosure would violate a state law that is more stringent than HIPAA, the information cannot be legally used or disclosed. The 12 public interest and benefit circumstances as well as the four other circumstances (TPO, disclosure to the individual, incidental uses and disclosures, and limited data sets) will be discussed in the following sections.

Public Interest and Benefit

The 12 public interest and benefit circumstances are detailed as follows. A use or disclosure may meet more than one of circumstances on the list.

1. *As required by law*: Disclosures are permitted when required by laws that meet the public interest requirements of disclosures relating to victims of abuse, neglect, or domestic violence; judicial and administrative proceedings; and law enforcement purposes.

2. *Public health activities:* Use or disclosure of PHI for public health activities serves such purposes as preventing or controlling diseases, injuries, and disabilities; reporting disease, injury (such as child abuse), and vital events such as births and deaths; and public health surveillance, investigation, or interventions.

   Examples include the reporting of adverse events or product defects in order to comply with Food and Drug Administration regulations and, when authorized by law, reporting a person who may have been exposed to a communicable disease and might be at risk for contracting or spreading it.

3. *Victims of abuse, neglect, or domestic violence:* An example is the reporting of a situation to authorities, such as Adult Protective Services, who are authorized by law to receive information about abuse or neglect. HIPAA does require the covered entity to promptly inform the individual that a report has been or will be made unless it believes doing so would place the individual at risk of serious harm if the covered entity would be informing the personal representative, whom it reasonably believes is responsible for the abuse, neglect, or other injury.

4. *Healthcare oversight activities:* An authorized health oversight agency may receive PHI under HIPAA for activities authorized by law, such as audits, civil or criminal investigations, licensure, and other inspections.

5. *Judicial and administrative proceedings:* Disclosures for judicial and administrative proceedings are permitted in response to an order of a court or an administrative tribunal, as long as the covered entity discloses only PHI expressly authorized by the order or other lawful process. For subpoenas and discovery requests, the party seeking the PHI must assure the covered entity it has made reasonable efforts to make the request known to the individual who is the subject of the PHI. In this situation, the entity must also be assured that the time for the individual to raise objections to the court or administrative tribunal has elapsed and that no objections were filed, all objections have been resolved, or a qualified protective order has been secured.

6. *Law enforcement purposes:* HIPAA lists six instances when disclosures to law enforcement do not require patient authorization or the opportunity to agree or object:

   a. Pursuant to legal process or otherwise required by law. Examples include a court order, court-ordered warrant, subpoena, or summons issued by a judicial officer. "As required by law" could be a law that requires reports of certain types of wounds or other physical injuries to law enforcement.

   b. In response to a law enforcement official's request to identify or locate a suspect, fugitive, material witness, or missing person. Only the following may be disclosed:

   ◆ Name and address

   ◆ Date and place of birth

   ◆ Social Security number

   ◆ ABO blood type and Rh factor

   ◆ Type of injury

   ◆ Date and time of treatment

   ◆ Date and time of death, if applicable

   ◆ Description of distinguishing physical characteristics, including height, weight, gender, race, hair and eye color, and presence or absence of facial scars or tattoos

c. In response to a law enforcement official's request about an individual who is or is suspected to be a victim of a crime (when the individual agrees to the disclosure or when the covered entity is unable to obtain the individual's agreement because of incapacity or emergency). The law enforcement official must represent that information is needed to determine whether a violation of law occurred, that immediate law enforcement activity depends on the disclosure, and disclosure is in the best interest of the individual as determined by the covered entity.

d. About a deceased individual when the covered entity suspects the death may have resulted from criminal conduct.

e. To a law enforcement official when the covered entity believes in good faith the information is evidence of criminal conduct that occurred on the covered entity's premises.

f. To a law enforcement official in response to a medical emergency when the covered entity believes disclosure is necessary to alert law enforcement to the commission and nature of a crime; the location or victims of such a crime; and the identity, description, and location of the perpetrator of such a crime. It is also permitted when the covered entity believes the medical emergency was the result of abuse, neglect, or domestic violence.

7. *Decedents:* HIPAA's privacy protections survive an individual's death, but disclosures to a coroner or medical examiner are permitted to identify a deceased person, determine a cause of death, or accomplish other purposes required by law. Disclosures to funeral directors are also permitted so they can carry out their duties. Information may be disclosed in reasonable anticipation of an individual's death.

8. *Cadaveric organ, eye, or tissue donation:* PHI may be disclosed to organ procurement agencies or other entities to facilitate the procurement, banking, or transplantation of cadaveric organs, eyes, or tissue.

9. *Research:* A covered entity may use or disclose PHI for research if an approved authorization waiver or alteration or other exceptions are met. Research is described more fully later in this chapter.

10. *Threat to health and safety:* Use and disclosure is allowed if the covered entity believes it is necessary to prevent or lessen a serious and imminent threat to the health or safety of an individual or the public. Disclosure must be made to a person who can reasonably prevent or lessen the threat. Disclosure is also permitted if necessary for law enforcement officials to apprehend an individual who may have caused harm to the victim or when it appears the individual has escaped from a correctional institution or lawful custody.

11. *Essential (specialized) government functions:* Uses and disclosures are permitted without authorization or the opportunity to agree or object as they relate to armed forces personnel for military and veterans activities, for purposes of national security and intelligence activities, for protective services for the President of the United States and others, and for public benefits and medical suitability determinations.

Disclosure of an inmate's PHI to correctional institutions or to a law enforcement official who has lawful custody is permitted if the correctional institution states the information is necessary to provide continuing healthcare; to secure the health and safety of the individual or other inmates, officers, employees, transportation personnel, or law enforcement on the premises; or to ensure administration and maintenance of the institution's safety, security, and good order.

12. *Workers' compensation:* Disclosure of PHI relating to work-related illness or injury, or workplace-related medical surveillance is permitted to the extent such disclosure complies with workers' compensation laws. (45 CFR 164.512)

TPO, To the Individual, Incidental Disclosures, Limited Data Sets

The four remaining circumstances where HIPAA permits PHI to be used or disclosed without either the individual's written authorization or an opportunity to agree or object are: TPO, disclosure to the individual, incidental uses and disclosures, and limited data sets. TPO refers collectively to a covered entity's functions that are necessary to successfully conduct business. HIPAA removes the authorization requirement for TPO because it would be too burdensome to require a written authorization each time PHI was needed to carry out these functions. Disclosure to the individual, discussed later in the chapter, refers to the right of access that HIPAA gives to individuals to obtain their own PHI. The final two circumstances are incidental uses and disclosures, and limited data sets.

Incidental uses and disclosures occur as part of doing business (45 CFR 164.502(a)(1)(iii)). An example would be calling out patients' names in a physician's office. As long as the information disclosed is the minimum necessary (for example, no diagnostic information is revealed), no authorization or opportunity to agree or object is required.

A **limited data set** is PHI that does not completely deidentify an individual, but eliminates most direct identifiers of the individual, the individual's relatives, employers, and household members. Deidentification restrictions are lifted for ages and dates, elements of geographic subdivisions (for example, postal address information cannot be included but town or city, state, and zip code can be included) and other unique identifying information (45 CFR 164.514(e)(2)). No authorization or opportunity to agree or object is required as long as the PHI is used or disclosed only for research, public health, or healthcare operations.

CHECK YOUR UNDERSTANDING 3.1

Instructions: Indicate whether the following statements are true or false (T or F).

1. The HIPAA consent explains an individual's rights and the covered entity's legal duties with respect to PHI.
2. The Notice of Privacy Practices must be presented to an individual upon each encounter with his healthcare provider.
3. Written authorization is required for an individual to be included in a facility directory.
4. One of the 12 public interest and benefit exceptions to the authorization requirements is disclosure to organ procurement agencies.
5. Incidental disclosures do not require an individual's written authorization.

Section 3: Preemption

When taking any action related to an individual's PHI that involves a state law, a covered entity must consider the legal concept of preemption. A covered entity has an obligation to comply with both state and federal laws; however, sometimes it is impossible to follow both. To address this conflict, the concept of **preemption** gives legal precedence to federal law. In other words, a covered entity must comply with the federal law when the federal and state laws conflict. There are some exceptions. If state law provides greater privacy protections or greater individual rights with regard to one's PHI (that is, it is more stringent), then state law will not be preempted by HIPAA.

There are also some other exceptions where state law will take precedence (that is, will not be preempted by HIPAA), even though it provides less privacy protection or lesser individual rights than HIPAA does. These exceptions are permitted because they serve an important public policy purpose such as regulating controlled substances. Other exceptions include laws that prevent healthcare fraud and abuse; regulate health plans; complete state reporting on healthcare delivery or costs; serve a compelling public health, safety or welfare need; provides for the reporting of vital statistics; and other public health data. It is important to review state legal requirements to determine whether state law or HIPAA prevails.

Section 4: Individual Rights

HIPAA gives individuals significant rights to allow some control over their PHI. Those rights are access, amendment, accounting of disclosures, restriction requests, and confidential communications. These rights are described in the following paragraphs and detailed in figure 3.7. Individuals also have the right to receive a NPP and to submit complaints when they believe HIPAA has been violated. Because covered entities are legally obligated to inform individuals about how to submit complaints, this is described under the "Administrative Requirements" later in the chapter.

Access

An individual has a right of **access** to inspect and obtain a copy of his or her own PHI that is in a designated record set (DRS), such as a health record (45 CFR 164.524). The individual's right extends for as long as the PHI is maintained.

Access to One's Own PHI

It is important that individuals generally be able to access their own PHI. Although the physical health record belongs to the organization that created it, the patient has an interest (or ownership) in his or her own information in the record. Without a specific right of access, providers and others can deny access. HITECH provides specific access requirements for electronic health records. These will be discussed in detail in chapter 6.

Per HIPAA, covered entities may require individuals to make their access requests in writing if it has informed them of this requirement. A covered entity must act on an individual's request within 30 days, and may extend the response just once by no more than 30 days as long as it responds within the initial 30-day window and gives the reason for the delay and a date by which it will respond.

FIGURE 3.7. | Individual Rights under HIPAA

Patient Rights at a Glance

Right	Request	Acceptance	Termination	Timeliness	Fee	Denial	Review
Right to request restriction of uses and disclosures	Provider must permit request, but does not have to be in writing.	Provider generally not required to agree, but if accepted, must not violate restriction except for emergency care. However, requests must be complied with (unless otherwise required by law) if disclosure would be to a health plan for payment or operations purposes and has been paid in full other than by the health plan.	Provider may terminate if individual agrees or requests in writing, or oral agreement is documented. Termination only applies to information created or received after the individual has been informed.	There is no provision for addressing timeliness.	There is no provision for a fee.	There are no requirements associated with denying restriction.	Not applicable
Right to receive confidential communications	Provider may require written request for receiving communications by alternative means or locations.	Provider must accommodate reasonable requests and may condition how payment will be handled but may not require explanation.	There is no provision for termination.	There is no provision for addressing timeliness.	There is no provision for a fee.	Not applicable	Not applicable

FIGURE 3.7. (Continued)

Patient Rights at a Glance

Right	Request	Acceptance	Termination	Timeliness	Fee	Denial	Review
Right of access to information	Provider must permit request for copying and inspection and may, upon notice, require requests in writing. Provider may supply a summary or explanation of information, instead, if individual agrees in advance.	Provider may deny access without opportunity for review if information is: psychotherapy notes, compiled for legal proceeding, subject to CLIA, about inmate and could cause harm, subject of research to which denial of access has been agreed, subject to Privacy Act, or obtained from someone else in confidence. Provider may deny access with opportunity to review if licensed professional determines access may endanger life or safety, there is reference to another person and access could cause harm, or request made by personal representative who may cause harm. Covered entities with EHRs must make information available electronically or must send it electronically upon the individual's request, in form and format requested (if readily producible as such).	Individuals have right of access for as long as information is maintained in designated record set.	Provider must act upon a request within 30 days, with one 30-day extension if individual is notified of reasons for delay and given date for access.	Provider may impose reasonable, cost-based fee for copying, postage, and preparing an explanation or summary.	If access is denied, provider must provide timely written explanation in plain language, containing basis for denial, review rights if applicable, description of how to file a complaint, and source of information not maintained by provider if known. Provider must also give individual access to any part of information not covered under grounds for denial.	An individual may request a review of a denial by a different healthcare professional.

(Continued on next page)

FIGURE 3.7. **(Continued)**

Patient Rights at a Glance

Right	Request	Acceptance	Termination	Timeliness	Fee	Denial	Review
Right to amend information	Provider must permit requests to amend a designated record set and may, upon notice, require request in writing and a reason.	If amendment is accepted, provider must append or link to record set and obtain and document identification and agreement to have provider notify relevant persons with which amendment needs to be shared. Provider may deny amendment if information was not created by the provider unless individual provides reasonable basis that originator is no longer available to act on request, is not part of designated record set, would not be available for access, or is accurate and complete.	Amendment applies for as long as information is maintained in designated record set.	Provider must act upon a request within 60 days of receipt. If unable to act on request within 60 days, provider may extend time by no more than 30 days provided individual is notified of reasons for delay and given date to amend.	There is no provision for a fee.	If amendment is denied, provider must provide timely written explanation in plain language, containing basis for denial, right to submit written statement of disagreement, right to request provider include request and denial with any future disclosures of information that is subject of amendment, and description of how to file a complaint.	Provider must accept written statement of disagreement (of limited length). Provider may prepare written rebuttal and must copy individual. Provider must append or link request, denial, disagreement, and rebuttal to record and include such or accurate summary with any subsequent disclosure. If no written disagreement, provider must include request and denial, or summary, in subsequent disclosures only if individual has requested such action.

FIGURE 3.7. (Continued)

Patient Rights at a Glance

Right	Request	Acceptance	Termination	Timeliness	Fee	Denial	Review
Right to accounting of disclosures	Provider must provide individual with written accounting including date of disclosure, name and address of recipient, description of information disclosed, purpose of disclosure or copy of individual's written authorization or other request for disclosure.	Provider must provide individual and retain documentation of written accounting of disclosures of PHI made in three years prior to date of request, except for disclosures (1) to carry out treatment, payment, and healthcare operations (this exception will not apply to covered entities with EHRs); (2) to the individuals themselves; (3) incident to a use or disclosure otherwise permitted or required; (4) pursuant to an authorization; (5) for the facility's director or to persons involved in the individual's care or other notification purposes; (6) for national security or intelligence purposes; (7) to correctional institutions or law enforcement as permitted; (8) as part of a limited data set; or (9) that occurred prior to the compliance date for the covered entity.	Not applicable	Provider must act upon request within 60 days of receipt. If unable to provide accounting, provider may extend time by no more than 30 days provided individual is notified of reasons for delay.	First accounting in any 12-month period must be provided without charge. A reasonable, cost-based fee may be charged for subsequent accountings in 12-month period if individual is notified in advance.	Provider must temporarily suspend right to receive an accounting of disclosures to health oversight agency or law enforcement official if agency or official provides written statement that accounting would impede their activities.	There is no provision for review of temporary suspension.

Adapted from Amatayakul 2001, AHIMA 2009, and AHIMA 2013.

A covered entity must arrange a convenient time and place of inspection with the individual or mail a copy of the PHI if the individual requests. PHI must be provided in the form or format requested if it can readily be produced that way. Otherwise, a readable hard-copy format or other mutually agreed-up format must be provided. A reasonable cost-based fee is permitted. Generally, fees may include:

- Copying, including supplies and labor
- Postage, when PHI is mailed
- Preparing an explanation or summary, if agreed to by the individual

Because retrieval fees cannot generally be attributed to the cost of providing PHI to an individual, they are not allowed under HIPAA. They are permissible for nonpatient requests.

Denial of Access without a Review

According to HIPAA, a covered entity can sometimes deny an individual access to PHI without giving an opportunity to review or appeal the denial.

Denials are not subject to an appeal if

- the PHI is in psychotherapy notes;
- information was compiled in reasonable anticipation of or use in a civil, criminal, or administrative action;
- PHI is maintained by a covered entity subject to the **Clinical Laboratory Improvements Amendments (CLIA) of 1988** (42 USC § 263a), if CLIA would prohibit access;
- PHI is maintained by a covered entity that is exempt from CLIA;
- the covered entity is a correctional institution or healthcare provider acting under a correctional institution's direction, and complying with an inmate's request would cause health or safety concerns;
- an individual, receiving treatment as part of a research study, agrees to suspend the right to access PHI temporarily (while the study is in progress);
- the PHI is contained in records that are subject to the federal Privacy Act (5 USC § 552a); or
- PHI was obtained from someone other than a healthcare provider under a promise of confidentiality and complying with the request would likely reveal the source of the information.

Denials must include a reason and tell the individual how he or she can complain to both the covered entity (with name and contact information provided) and the Secretary of HHS.

Denial of Access with a Review

HIPAA requires an individual be given the right to review a denial when a licensed healthcare professional determines that access to requested PHI would

- likely endanger the life or physical safety of the individual or another person, or
- reasonably endanger the life or physical safety of another person mentioned in the PHI

When a reviewable denial is made, the individual must be told that he or she has the right to request a review of the denial. This must be conducted by a licensed healthcare professional who was not involved in the original decision. The covered entity must grant or deny access according to the reviewing official's decision. Reviewable denials must also include a reason and tell the individual how he or she can complain to both the covered entity (with name and contact information provided) and the Secretary of HHS.

Amendment

HIPAA permits an individual to request that a covered entity make an **amendment** to PHI in a DRS (45 CFR 164.526). However, the covered entity may deny the request if it determines that the PHI or the record

- was not created by the covered entity;
- is not part of the DRS;
- is not available for inspection per access restrictions (for example, psychotherapy notes); or
- is accurate and complete.

The covered entity may require a written amendment request and provide a reason for requesting the amendment. This requirement must be communicated in advance to the individual, usually in the NPP.

A covered entity must act on an individual's amendment request within 60 days by granting it or denying it in writing. It may extend the response just once by no more than 30 days if the reason for the delay is explained in writing and a completion date is given.

If a covered entity grants an amendment request, it must

1. identify the records in the DRS that are affected by the amendment and append the information or give the link to the amendment's location; and
2. inform the individual that the amendment was accepted, have him or her identify the persons with whom the amendment needs to be shared, and obtain his or her agreement to notify those persons. The covered entity must make reasonable efforts to provide the amendment within a reasonable amount of time to anyone who has received the PHI, as well as those relying on the corrected information.

Denials of amendment requests must be written in plain language and contain

- the basis for the denial;
- the individual's right to submit a written statement disagreeing with the denial;
- the process to submit the disagreement;
- a statement explaining how, if the individual does not submit a disagreement to the denial, he or she may request that both the original amendment request and the covered entity's denial accompany any future disclosures of the PHI that is the subject of the amendment; and
- a description of how the individual may complain to the covered entity (with name and contact information provided). (45 CFR 164.526(d))

The covered entity may write a rebuttal to individual's disagreement, providing the individual with a copy.

If an individual writes a disagreement, the amendment request, denial, individual's disagreement, and rebuttal (if one was created) must be appended or linked to the subject record or PHI. When future disclosures of the information are made, this material or a summary of it must accompany it. However, if an individual did not write a disagreement to the covered entity's denial, the amendment request and denial must only accompany future disclosures if the individual requests it.

Accounting of Disclosures

Maintaining a procedure to track PHI disclosures has been a common practice in departments that manage health information. However, HIPAA provides for an **accounting of disclosures** that gives an individual the right to receive a list of certain disclosures that a covered entity has made (45 CFR 164.528).

Disclosures for which an accounting is not required include:

- TPO (although this exception is only applicable to covered entities without EHRs per HITECH)
- To the individual to whom the information pertains
- Incidental to an otherwise permitted or required use or disclosure
- Pursuant to an authorization
- For use in the facility's directory, to persons involved in the individual's care, or for other notification purposes
- To meet national security or intelligence requirements
- To correctional institutions or law enforcement officials
- As part of a limited data set
- Disclosures that occurred before the HIPAA compliance date (45 CFR 164.528)

The accounting requirement includes disclosures made in writing, electronically, by telephone, or orally. The 12 public interest and benefit circumstances described in the previous section about authorizations must be included in an accounting. Erroneous disclosures (such as a facsimile transmitted to the wrong recipient) are also subject to the accounting requirement. It does not matter whether the recipient read the information. Erroneous disclosures may also constitute breaches. One activity that appears to be a healthcare operation, but is not, is mandatory public health reporting such as the reporting of births, deaths, and communicable diseases. Where TPO must be disclosed (by covered entities with EHRs, per HITECH), this distinction is not important. However, the distinction is important for paper-based and oral disclosures.

The individual's right to an accounting may be suspended at the written request of a health oversight agency or law enforcement official as long as a written request indicates that an accounting would impede its activities. The request must also state how long a suspension is required.

Items that must be included in an accounting are the date of disclosure, name and address (when known) of the entity or person who received the information, a brief description of the PHI disclosed, and a brief statement of the purpose of the disclosure or a copy of the request for an disclosure. Originally, the accounting had to address disclosures during the previous six years. This was revised per HITECH.

A covered entity must act on a request within 60 days but may extend it, just once, by no more than 30 days as long as it notifies the individual in writing of the reasons for the delay and when the accounting will be made available. A proposed administrative rule issued by HHS on May 31, 2011, after HITECH was published, suggests decreasing the 60-day time period. The first accounting within any 12-month period must be provided without charge. Subsequent requests within a 12-month period may result in a reasonable cost-based fee as long as the individual is informed in advance and given the opportunity to withdraw or modify the request. Documentation must be maintained on all accounting requests, including the information in the accounting, the written accounting that was provided to the individual, and the titles of persons or offices responsible for receiving and processing requests for an accounting. Policies and procedures must be developed to ensure that PHI disclosed from all areas of an organization, especially those areas outside a health information management (HIM) department, can be tracked and compiled when an accounting request is received.

As mentioned previously, HITECH made some revisions to the accounting requirement. Additionally, in the May 31, 2011 proposed administrative rule, further changes to the accounting requirement were proposed. One of these, the proposed addition on an access report, was substantial. This will be discussed in detail in chapter 6.

Restriction Requests

Per HIPAA, a covered entity must permit an individual to make a **restriction request** regarding uses and disclosures of PHI for carrying out TPO (45 CFR 164.522(a)(1)). Generally, a covered entity has discretion to agree or not agree to a request. In some cases, it may not be allowed to honor a request (for example, where disclosures are required by law). If it agrees, however, it must abide by it. The restriction can be terminated by either the individual or by the covered entity. When the covered entity initiates termination, it must inform the individual. The termination is only effective with respect to the PHI created or received after the individual has been informed (45 CFR 164.522(a)(1)). HITECH creates one exception where a covered entity must agree to restriction requests. This is outlined in figure 3.7 and is explained further in Chapter 6.

Confidential Communications

Healthcare providers and health plans must give individuals the right of **confidential communications**, or the opportunity to request that communications of PHI be routed to an alternative location or by an alternative method (45 CFR 164.522(b)(1)). Healthcare providers must honor a request without a reason if the request is reasonable. Health plans must honor requests that are reasonable, but may require a statement that disclosure could pose a safety risk. Both healthcare providers and health plans may refuse to accommodate a request if the individual does not provide information as to how payment will be handled or if the individual does not provide an alternative address or method by which he or she can be contacted.

An example of a request for confidential communications would be a woman who requests that billing information from her psychiatrist, from whom she is seeking treatment because of domestic violence, be sent to her work address instead of to her home.

CHECK YOUR UNDERSTANDING 3.2

Instructions: Indicate whether the following statements are true or false (T or F).

1. A covered entity must act on an accounting of disclosures request within 60 days with one 30-day extension permitted.
2. A covered entity may deny an amendment request if it determines that it is not part of the DRS.
3. For confidential communications requests, a health plan may require a statement that disclosure could pose a safety risk.
4. A denial of access is not subject to appeal if access was denied because PHI was obtained from someone other than a healthcare provider under a promise of confidentiality and complying with the request would likely reveal the source of the information.
5. The concept of preemption gives legal precedence to state law.

Section 5: Marketing and Fundraising

Marketing

HIPAA defines **marketing** as a communication about a product or service that encourages the recipient to purchase or use that product or service (45 CFR 164.501). As a general HIPAA rule, an individual's authorization must be obtained prior to using his or her PHI for marketing. However, marketing has posed some difficulty because covered entities have classified marketing activities as a healthcare operation, either mistakenly or to avoid the authorization requirement.

Per HIPAA, certain communications look like marketing but, by definition, are not. Instead, they are considered healthcare operations and do not require an authorization. They are communications that

- describe a health-related product or service (or payment for the product or service) provided by or included in the benefit plan of the covered entity making the communication, including communications about participants in the healthcare provider's or health plan's network;
- describe replacements or enhancements to a health plan;
- describe available health-related products or services available to a health plan enrollee that are of value, although not part of a benefit plan;
- provide refill reminders or otherwise communicate about a drug or biologic that is currently being prescribed for the individual, when the remuneration is reasonably related to the cost of making the communication;

- are for treatment of the individual; and
- are for case management or care coordination for the individual, or to direct or recommend alternative treatments, therapies, healthcare providers, or settings of care. (45 CFR 164.501)

Common communications that meet the marketing definition of marketing but do not require authorization are those that

- occur face-to-face between the covered entity and the individual (not including communications via phone, mail, or e-mail, which *do* require an authorization) or
- concern a promotional gift of nominal value provided by the covered entity (45 CFR 164.508(a)(3)).

HITECH has strengthened what is considered marketing.

Fundraising

For **fundraising** activities that benefit a covered entity, HIPAA permits the covered entity to use or disclose to a BA or an institutionally related foundation, without authorization, demographic information and dates of healthcare provided to an individual (45 CFR 164.514(f)). Individuals must be informed in the NPP that PHI may be used for this purpose. Fundraising materials must include instructions on how to opt out of receiving solicitations in the future. If the individual has opted out of fundraising, this is to be treated as a revocation and no further solicitations may be sent to that individual. Fundraising may target a department of service or treating physician. However, if a fundraising activity targets individuals based on diagnosis (for example, patients with kidney disease are targeted to raise funds for a new kidney dialysis center), prior authorization is required. HITECH has strengthened fundraising requirements.

Section 6: Research

Human subjects have been misused historically in research activities. Because of this, there are many controls on human subject research. In addition to other regulations listed below, HIPAA provides some controls.

The Federal Policy for the Protection of Human Subjects (the Common Rule) was developed from the joint creation of regulations from several federal agencies and, specifically, from HHS regulations. In 1991, the portion of the HHS regulations that focused on the protection of human subjects (45 CFR Part 46(a)) was adopted by a number of federal departments and agencies that either conducted or funded human subject research. Requirements of the Common Rule include:

- Compliance assurances by organizations conducting research
- Informed consent
- Special protections for vulnerable populations such as prisoners, pregnant women, children, mentally disabled persons, and economically or educationally disadvantaged persons (45 CFR 46.101–46.112)

Additionally, an **institutional review board (IRB)** must approve federally funded human subject research, even if the patient has signed an informed consent.

HIPAA provides additional protections where research places human subjects and their private information at risk. It requires generally that authorization must be obtained for uses and disclosures of PHI created as part of research (AHIMA 2011c). Whereas the Common Rule regulates only federally funded research, HIPAA regulates both privately and federally funded research. As a result, covered entities must create privacy boards if IRBs do not already exist (Amatayakul 2003). A **privacy board** is a group formed by a covered entity to review research studies where authorization waivers are requested and to ensure the HIPAA privacy rights of research subjects. In addition to the privacy board requirement, HIPAA addresses when an authorization for use and disclosure of PHI is required from an individual, and in what form the authorization may occur.

HIPAA (CFR 164.508(b)(4)) has generally prohibited covered entities from using **conditioned authorizations**, which make treatment, payment, and health plan enrollment or benefit eligibility contingent on an individual signing an authorization, unless it was for purposes such as treatment-related research and health plan enrollment. This was to discourage coercing individuals to sign an authorization in order to receive services. Consequently, **compound authorizations** (which combine informed consent with an authorization to use or disclose PHI) have been limited, and **stand-alone authorizations**, which include the core elements of a valid authorization (45 CFR 164.508), have been preferred. HITECH has made some concessions regarding the combination of conditioned and **unconditioned authorizations** for research.

In a blinded study, or where there is minimal risk to the individual's privacy (for example, research limited to health record reviews), a **waived authorization** (that is, no individual authorization) or **altered authorization** (that is, one or more of the authorization requirements have been changed per approval of the IRB or privacy board, but authorization is still required) may be permitted (45 CFR 164.512). HIPAA also permits waiver of authorization where the researcher provides assurance that

- the use or disclosure of PHI is solely preparatory to the research itself, and it will not be removed from the covered entity;
- the use or disclosure is solely for research on decedents' PHI; or
- only a limited data set will be used for research, public health, or healthcare operations, and a limited data set use agreement is in place. (45 CFR 164.512(i))

A limited data set is PHI that does not completely deidentify an individual, but eliminates most direct identifers of the individual, the individual's relatives, employers, and household members (45 CFR 164.514(e)(2)). If deidentified information or a limited data set is used for research, an accounting of disclosures is not required. HIPAA imposes many requirements on research activities. Figure 3.8 provides an analysis of the responsibilities of the IRB and the researcher under HIPAA (Amatayakul 2003).

FIGURE 3.8.	Actions required for use of PHI in research

Actions Required by HIPAA for Use of PHI in Research

Type of Information	IRB	Researcher	Research Subject (patient or decedent)
PHI preparatory to research	None*	Representation that use is solely and necessary for research and will not be removed from covered entity	None
Deidentified health information	None*	Removal of safe-harbor data or statistical assurance of deidentification	None
Limited data set	None*	Removal of direct identifiers and data use agreement	None
Individually identifiable on health information on decedents	None*	Representation that use is solely and necessary for research on decedents and documentation of death upon request of covered entity	None
PHI of human subjects (whether research is interventional or record review)	Waive authorization requirement if determined that risk to privacy is minimal	Representation that: 1. Privacy risk is minimal based on: • plan to protect identifiers • plan to destroy identifiers unless there is a health or research reason to retain • written assurance that PHI will not be reused or redisclosed 2. Research requires use of specifically described PHI 3. Justify the waiver 4. Obtain IRB approval under normal or expedited review procedures	None

(Continued on next page)

FIGURE 3.8.	(Continued)		
	Actions Required by HIPAA for Use of PHI in Research		
Type of Information	IRB	Researcher	Research Subject (patient or decedent)
	Approve alteration of authorization (for example, to restrict patient's access during study) if determined that risk to privacy is minimal	Same as above	Sign altered authorization form
	Approve research protocol ensuring that there is an authorization for use either combined with consent for and disclosure of PHI research or separate		Sign authorization combined with consent for research or sign standard authorization for use and disclosure of PHI for research as described in authorization

*There may be requirements imposed by the IRB, but there are none imposed by HIPAA.

Source: Amatayakul 2003

Section 7: Administrative Requirements

HIPAA imposes important administrative requirements including:

- Standards for policies and procedures and changes to policies and procedures
- Designation of a privacy officer and a contact person for receiving complaints
- Requirements for workforce privacy training
- Requirements for sanctions
- Mitigation of wrongful use and disclosure
- Requirements for establishing data safeguards
- A process for individuals to submit complaints
- Prohibition against retaliation and waiver
- Requirements for documentation retention (45 CFR 164.530)

Policies and Procedures

A covered entity must implement policies and procedures to ensure compliance with all aspects of HIPAA. Privacy policies and procedures must be routinely reviewed, and changes must be made to be consistent with changes in the privacy and security regulations (45 CFR 164.530(i)). Any regulatory changes that materially affect the NPP must be updated in the NPP.

Privacy Officer and Contact Person

HIPAA requires that covered entities designate an individual—a **privacy officer**—to be responsible for developing and implementing privacy policies and procedures. Additionally, the covered entity must designate a person as responsible for receiving complaints. This individual must be able to provide further information about matters covered by the entity's NPP (45 CFR 164.530(a)).

Workforce Training

Every member of a covered entity's **workforce** must be trained in PHI policies and procedures. New members must be trained within a reasonable period of time after joining the workforce. All workforce members must receive updated training when material changes are made to policies or procedures regarding privacy (45 CFR 164.530(b)). Workforce training should be comprehensive, including those not employed by the covered entity and those who do not work directly with PHI but who may nonetheless come into contact with it (for example, outsourced vendors' employees who work routinely on the covered entity's premises and custodial staff). BAs should also train their workforce members because of the heightened liability for BAs under HITECH.

Documentation must be maintained as evidence that privacy training has occurred. Although not required, a signed statement of training by each workforce member would be helpful in documenting compliance. The covered entity should document all steps that have been taken to ensure—to the extent possible—compliance by its workforce. In addition to documentation to support workforce attendance at training sessions, workforce members should sign nondisclosure agreements confirming their understanding of HIPAA and commitment to protecting the privacy of patient information.

Sanctions

Covered entities are required to establish sanctions for noncompliance with HIPAA and the organization's accompanying privacy policies and procedures (45 CFR 164.530(e)). The sanctions must be applied against workforce members who do not comply with HIPAA or the policies and procedures the covered entity has put in place.

Mitigation

HIPAA requires covered entities to mitigate, as much as possible, harmful effects that result from the wrongful use and disclosure of PHI (45 CFR 164.530(f)). **Mitigation** is the lessening of negative consequences. Although HITECH has forced one type of mitigation—breach notification—other types of mitigation may assuage the individual, including:

- Apology
- Disciplinary action against the responsible employee or employees (although such results will not be able to be shared with the wronged individual)

- Repair of the process that resulted in the breach
- Payment of a bill or financial loss that resulted from the infraction
- Gestures of goodwill and good public relations (such as awarding gift certificates) (AHIMA 2010)

Mitigation may result from discovery of a breach by a covered entity or BA, or from a complaint that an individual has filed with the organization, the **Office for Civil Rights (OCR)** for HHS, or both. Determining when the individual should be informed and what other steps should be taken can be difficult for an organization. Policies and procedures, followed by complete and detailed documentation when a situation arises, are critical to a successful mitigation process (AHIMA 2010).

Data Safeguards

Covered entities must have appropriate administrative, technical, and physical safeguards in place to protect the privacy of PHI from intentional and unintentional uses or disclosures that violate HIPAA. These safeguards must limit incidental uses and disclosures (45 CFR 164.530(c)). Examples include shredding paper documents containing PHI and limiting access to areas containing PHI through the use of devices such as keycards, passwords, or locks.

Complaints

A covered entity must provide a way for an individual to complain about the entity's policies and procedures, noncompliance with policies and procedures, or alleged HIPAA violations. The NPP must contain contact information about the covered entity and inform individuals that they may submit complaints to the OCR (45 CFR 164.530(d)). The OCR has regional offices that field complaints from individuals in that region. The covered entity must document all complaints and the disposition of each complaint.

Retaliation and Waiver

To not deter individuals from exercising their right to complain about alleged HIPAA violations, covered entities are prohibited from **retaliation and waiver**. Covered entities may not retaliate against anyone who exercises his or her rights under HIPAA, assists in an investigation by HHS or another appropriate investigative authority, or opposes an act or practice that the person believes is a HIPAA violation (45 CFR 164.530(g)). Further, individuals cannot be required to waive their HIPAA rights to obtain treatment, payment, or enrollment and benefits eligibility (45 CFR 164.530(h)).

Documentation and Record Retention

Six years is the period for which HIPAA-related documents must be retained. This timeframe refers to the latter of the following: the date the document was created or the last effective date of the document (45 CFR 164.530(j)). Documents affected by this requirement include policies and procedures, the NPP, complaint dispositions, and other actions, activities, and designations that HIPAA requires to be documented.

REAL-WORLD CASE

In Indiana, a medical practice referred a patient's case to a collections agency for nonpayments. When records were sent to the collections agency, staff at the medical practice failed to remove highly sensitive information about the patient's HIV status. The records became evidence in a court action where collection was pursued. As part of the court case, the patient's HIV status became public record. The patient sued and won $1.25 million in damages.

Individuals are not able to sue using HIPAA as a legal theory that forms the basis of a lawsuit (that is, a cause of action). Instead this individual filed his lawsuit under Indiana's medical malpractice act. Lawsuits stemming from the wrongful disclosure of patient information are generally based on tort (civil wrong) theories such as negligence or invasion of privacy. Negligence is a very broad cause of action that can apply to many types of cases. As long as all of the required elements, or parts, of negligence are met (duty to the patient, breach of the duty, causation, and harm), an individual may have a successful lawsuit.

This case provides a good reminder that a patient's recourse for a HIPAA violation is currently limited to filing complaints with the OCR for the Department of Health and Human Services (HHS). Any fines or settlement amounts received are retained by OCR.

HITECH has added remedies such as enabling state Attorneys General to file lawsuits on behalf of their citizens based on alleged HIPAA violations. Also, individual compensation has been proposed as a way to make a person whole after he or she has been harmed by a HIPAA violation. A few lawsuits have been filed by state Attorneys General, as will be discussed in chapter 6. However, individual compensation has not yet occurred (AHIMA 2011a).

SUMMARY

The HIPAA Privacy and Security Rules act together to regulate the privacy and security of patient information. The Privacy Rule applies to all forms of PHI. This chapter discussed HIPAA Privacy Rule requirements by focusing on key documents; situations where patient authorization is and is not required prior to PHI being used or disclosed; the preemption doctrine; individual rights; parameters surrounding the use and disclosure of PHI for marketing, fundraising, and research; and administrative requirements.

REFERENCES

Amatayakal, M. 2003. HIPAA on the job: Another layer of regulations: Research under HIPAA. *Journal of AHIMA* 74(1):16A–16D.

Amatayakal, M. 2001. HIPAA on the job: Managing individual rights requirements under HIPAA privacy. *Journal of AHIMA* 72(6):16A–16D.

American Health Information Management Association. 2013. Analysis of Modifications to the HIPAA Privacy, Security, Enforcement, and Breach Notification Rules Under the Health Information Technology for Economic and Clinical Health Act and the Genetic Nondiscrimination Act; Other Modifications to the HIPAA Rules. http://library.ahima.org/xpedio/groups/public/documents/ahima/bok1_050067.pdf.

American Health Information Management Association. 2012a. Appendix A: Authorization checklist—required elements. *Journal of AHIMA* 83(2): expanded online version. http://library.ahima.org/xpedio/groups/public/documents/ahima/bok1_049362.hcsp?dDocName=bok1_049362.

American Health Information Management Association. 2012b. Appendix B: Sample authorization to disclose health information. *Journal of AHIMA* 83(2). http://library.ahima.org/xpedio/groups/public/documents/ahima/bok1_049363.hcsp?dDocName=bok1_049363.

American Health Information Management Association. 2011a. HIPAA violation? Sue me. *Journal of AHIMA* 82(3): 68.

American Health Information Management Association. 2011b. *Notice of Privacy Practices* (Updated). Appendix A: Sample Notice of Privacy Practices. Chicago: AHIMA.

American Health Information Management Association. 2011c. Regulations Governing Research. http://library.ahima.org/xpedio/idcplg?IdcService=GET_HIGHLIGHT_INFO&QueryText=%28Regulations+Governing+Research%29%3cand%3e%28xPublishSite%3csubstring%3e%60BoK%60%29&SortField=xPubDate&SortOrder=Desc&dDocName=bok1_048639&HighlightType=HtmlHighlight&dWebExtension=hcsp.

American Health Information Management Association, American Medical Informatics Association. 2010. Handling complaints and mitigation (Updated). *Journal of AHIMA* http://library.ahima.org/xpedio/groups/public/documents/ahima/bok1_047811.hcsp?dDocName=bok1_047811.

Brodnik, M., L. Rinehart-Thompson, and R. Reynolds. 2012. *Fundamentals of Law for Health Informatics and Information Management*. Chicago: AHIMA.

Department of Health and Human Services. 2010. Modifications to the HIPAA Privacy, Security, and Enforcement Rules under the Health Information Technology for Economic and Clinical Health Act; Proposed Rule. 45 CFR Parts 160 and 164. *Federal Register* 75(134): 40868-40924.

Department of Health and Human Services. 2002. Standards for Privacy of Individually Identifiable Health Information; Security Standards for the Protection of Electronic Protected Health

Information; General Administrative Requirements Including Civil Monetary Penalties: Procedures for Investigations, Imposition of Penalties, and Hearings. Final Rule. 45 CFR Parts 160 and 164. *Federal Register* 67(157): 53181-53273.

Department of Health and Human Services. 2003. Must an Authorization Include an Expiration Date? http://www.hhs.gov/hipaafaq/use/476.html.

45 CFR Part 46a: Basic HHS Policy for Protection of Human Research Subjects. 2005.

45 CFR 46.101–46.112: Protection of Human Subjects. 2005.

45 CFR 164.501: Definitions. 2006.

45 CFR 164.502(a)(1)(iii)): Incidental uses and disclosures. 2006.

45 CFR 164.506(b): Consent for uses and disclosures permitted. 2006.

45 CFR 164.508: Uses and disclosures for which an authorization is required. 2006.

45 CFR 164.508(a)(2): Authorization required: psychotherapy notes. 2006.

45 CFR 164.508(a)(3): Authorization required: marketing. 2006.

45 CFR 164.508(b)(2): Defective authorizations. 2006.

45 CFR 164.508(b)(4): Prohibition on conditioning of authorizations. 2006.

45 CFR §164.508(c): Implementation specifications: Core elements and requirements. 2006.

45 CFR 164.510: Uses and disclosures requiring an opportunity for the individual to agree or to object. 2006.

45 CFR 164.510(b): Standard: uses and disclosures for involvement in the individual's care and notification purposes. 2006.

45 CFR 164.512: Uses and disclosures for which an authorization or opportunity to agree or object it not required. 2006.

45 CFR 164.512(i): Standard: uses and disclosures for research purposes. 2006.

45 CFR 164.514(e)(2): Implementation specification: limited data set. 2006.

45 CFR 164.514(f): Standard: uses and disclosures for fundraising. 2006.

45 CFR 164.520: Notice of privacy practices for protected health information. 2006.

45 CFR 164.520(c)(2): Specific requirements for certain covered healthcare providers. 2006.

45 CFR 164.522(a)(1): Standard: right of an individual to request restriction of uses and disclosures. 2006.

45 CFR 164.522(b)(1): Standard: confidential communications requirements. 2006.

45 CFR 164.524: Access of individuals to protected health information. 2006.

45 CFR 164.526: Amendment to protected health information. 2006.

45 CFR 164.526(d): Implementation specifications; denying the amendment. 2006.

45 CFR 164.528: Accounting of disclosures of protected health information. 2006.

45 CFR 164.530: Administrative requirements. 2006.

45 CFR 164.530(a): Standard: personnel designations. 2006.

45 CFR 164.530(b): Standard: training. 2006.

45 CFR 164.530(c): Standard: safeguards. 2006.

45 CFR 164.530(d): Standard: complaints to the covered entity. 2006.

45 CFR 164.530(e): Standard: sanctions. 2006.

45 CFR 164.530(f): Standard: mitigation. 2006.

45 CFR 164.530(g): Standard: refraining from intimidating or retaliatory acts. 2006.

CFR 164.530(h): Standard: waiver of rights. 2006.

45 CFR 164.530(i): Standard: policies and procedures. 2006.

45 CFR 164.530(j): Standard: documentation. 2006.

5 USC §552a: The privacy act of 1974.

CHAPTER **4**

HIPAA Security Rule Concepts

Learning Objectives

- Explain differences between the HIPAA Security Rule and the HIPAA Privacy Rule

- Explain how the requirements of the HIPAA Security Rule can be applied to organizations of varying sizes and varying levels of technical sophistication

- Distinguish required and addressable implementation specifications

- Describe the purpose of physical safeguards; list the four safeguards and identify their implementation specifications

- Describe the purpose of technical safeguards; list the five safeguards and identify their implementation specifications

- Describe the purpose of administrative safeguards; list the nine safeguards and identify their implementation specifications

- Describe the purpose of the Security Rule's organizational requirements; list the two requirements and identify their implementation specifications

- Describe the purpose of the Security Rule's policies and procedures and documentation requirements; list the two policies and procedures and documentation requirements and identify their implementation specifications

KEY TERMS

Account lockout

Addressable specification

Administrative safeguards

Antivirus software packages

Audit controls

Audit log

Audit trail

Authentication

"Break the glass"

Context-based access control (CBAC)

Contingency plan

Cryptography

Decryption

Electronic protected health information (ePHI)

Encryption

Entity authentication

Firewall

Flexible

Full disk encryption

Implementation specification

Integrity

Intrusion detection systems

Intrusion prevention systems

Invalid log-on attempt

Metadata

Person authentication

Physical safeguards

Private key infrastructure (PKI)

Public key infrastructure

Required specification

Risk management

Role-based access control (RBAC)

Scalable

Self-encrypted hard drives

Single-factor authentication

Technical safeguards

Technology neutral

Transmission security

Two-factor authentication

User-based access control (UBAC)

Workstation

INTRODUCTION

The HIPAA Security Rule regulates the maintenance and transmission of **electronic protected health information (ePHI)**, which is individually identifiable health information created or received electronically by a covered entity or business associate (AHIMA 2012). The scope of the Security Rule contrasts with the HIPAA Privacy Rule, which regulates all types of PHI (including paper, electronic, and oral) rather than applying to ePHI only. Because of its application to ePHI, the Security Rule places a greater emphasis on technology. Additionally, the Security Rule's focus is limited to the obligations of covered entities and business associates in safeguarding ePHI. The Privacy Rule, however, also emphasizes the rights of individuals regarding their own health information.

Covered entities originally were required to comply with the Security Rule beginning April 21, 2005. The compliance deadline was delayed until April 21, 2006 for small health plans. As will be discussed further in chapter six, the Health Information Technology for Economic and Clinical Health (HITECH) Act of the American Recovery and Reinvestment Act (ARRA) also requires business associates (BAs) to comply with the Security Rule. This chapter will introduce the reader to the Security Rule's required administrative, physical, and technical safeguards as well as organizational requirements and standards for policies, procedures, and documentation. The security standards are located at 45 CFR 164.302 through 45 CFR164.318.

Section 1: General Concepts and Definitions

The Security Rule requires that covered entities do four things:

1. Ensure confidentiality, integrity, and availability of all electronic PHI (ePHI) created, received, maintained, or transmitted

2. Protect against reasonably anticipated threats or hazards that might affect the security of integrity of ePHI

3. Protect against reasonably anticipated uses or disclosures of ePHI that is not permitted or required

4. Ensure workforce compliance (45 CFR 164.306(a))

The Security Rule is flexible, scalable, and technology neutral. **Flexible** means that a covered entity is permitted to use any security measures that allow it to reasonably and appropriately implement the standards and implementation specifications (45 CFR 164.306(b)). However, when deciding what security measures to take, organizations must consider their

- Size, complexity, and capabilities
- Technical infrastructure, hardware, and software security capabilities
- Cost of security measures
- Probability and criticality of potential risks to ePHI (45 CFR 164.306(b))

Scalable means that it is written to accommodate and apply to organizations of any size. **Technology neutral** means that it does not require or prescribe certain technologies. Rather, it allows organizations to develop as their individual technological capabilities allow and holds organizations accountable to comply with the rule.

The Security Rule consists of five categories of standards:

1. Physical safeguards (45 CFR 164.310)
2. Technical safeguards (45 CFR 164.312)
3. Administrative safeguards (45 CFR 164.308)
4. Organizational requirements (45 CFR 164.314)
5. Policies and procedures and documentation requirements (45 CFR 164.316)

Implementation specifications, which provide further detailed instructions for how the standards should be carried out, are either "required" or "addressable" (45 CFR 164.306(d)). A **required specification** is mandatory and must be implemented for compliance. An **addressable specification** is met if the organization:

- Determines the specification is reasonable and appropriate, so it implements it as written

- Determines the specification is not reasonable and appropriate, so it implements a reasonable and appropriate equivalent alternative, or documents why it would not be reasonable and appropriate to implement it (45 CFR 164.306(d))

One reason a specification may not be reasonable and appropriate to implement is if the risk for which the specification was written does not exist or there is a negligible likelihood of it occurring. One should not be misled into thinking that addressable specifications are optional, however. They are not optional and they cannot be disregarded. If they are not implemented, complete documentation must be present to justify the lack of implementation.

Section 2: Physical Safeguards

Physical safeguards are "physical measures, policies, and procedures to protect a covered entity's electronic information systems and related buildings and equipment, from natural and environmental hazards, and unauthorized intrusion" (45 CFR 164.304).

The four physical safeguard standards are listed in 45 CFR 164.310. They are outlined in figure 4.1. The implementation specifications within each standard are identified as either required or addressable. Standards 2 and 3, Workstation Use and Workstation Security, do not have implementation specifications.

Facility Access Controls (45 CFR 164.310(a)(1))

Facility access controls (four implementation specifications, all addressable) require that limits be placed on physical access to electronic information systems and the facilities in which they are located. At the same time, properly authorized access must be permitted. The Security Rule defines facility as the physical premises and the interior and exterior of buildings (45 CFR 164.304). All locations where there is physical access to ePHI must be considered including the homes of workforce members and other physical locations (HHS 2007b).

Contingency Operations (45 CFR 164.310(a)(2)(i))

The first implementation specification, contingency operations (addressable), states that if there is an emergency, procedures are to be established to allow the facility to access and restore lost data as part of a disaster recovery plan and emergency mode of operations plan. These procedures may be implemented during or immediately after a disaster or emergency and must be carried out to ensure both security and appropriate access of ePHI (HHS 2007b).

FIGURE 4.1.	Physical safeguard standards		
Standards	**Sections**	**Implementation Specifications** **(R) = Required, (A) = Addressable**	
Facility Access Controls	§ 164.310(a)(1)	Contingency Operations	**(A)**
		Facility Security Plan	**(A)**
		Access Control and Validation Procedures	**(A)**
		Maintenance Records	**(A)**
Workstation Use	§ 164.310(b)		
Workstation Security	§ 164.310(c)		
Device and Media Controls	§ 164.310(d)(1)	Disposal	**(R)**
		Media Reuse	**(R)**
		Accountability	**(A)**
		Data Backup and Storage	**(A)**

Source: HHS 2007b

Facility Security Plan (45 CFR 164.310(a)(2)(ii))

The second implementation specification, facility security plan (addressable), calls for policies and procedures to protect a facility and its equipment from unauthorized physical access, including tampering and theft. Although data protection is critical, appropriate access to those with legitimate business needs also must be facilitated. For example, the needs of staff, patients, visitors, and business partners to access facilities and equipment must be addressed. Common controls that help prevent unauthorized physical access include locked doors, signs warning of restricted access, surveillance cameras and alarms. Movable property may be controlled through the use of property control tags or engraving. Personnel may be controlled through staff or visitor identification badges as well as security escorts. An organization may also hire or contract security services to patrol the premises. Workforce members should know the roles they play in ensuring facility security (HHS 2007b).

Access Control and Validation Procedures (45 CFR 164.310(a)(2)(iii))

The third implementation specification, access control and validation procedures (addressable), states that procedures are to be implemented that both control and validate a person's access to facilities. The level of access is to be based on an individual's role or function within the organization, including control of visitor access and control over access to software programs for testing and revision. Access control and validation is closely linked to the facility security plan (HHS 2007b).

Role-based access control (RBAC) gives access to users based on their roles as members of the organization. Users are assigned to pre-established groups with certain access privileges based on the group's need to access the information. For example, Ellen is a nurse and authorized user at Township Hospital. As a result, she is placed in a group that gives her access to the clinical components of the system relevant to her role. This type of access control can be compared to two other types: user-based access control and context-based access control. **User-based access control (UBAC)**, grants access to users based on their individual identity. For example, Ellen may be given access because she is an authorized user in Township Hospital's information system. **Context-based access control (CBAC)** is the most stringent mechanism. It limits users' access to information based not only on their identity and role, but also their location and the time of access (AHIMA 2012). For example, under CBAC Ellen is a nurse and authorized system user and, as such, is given access to the clinical components of the system relevant to her role. However, because CBAC also considers the context of access, she may only access information from 7:00 a.m. to 7:00 p.m. on Saturdays and Sundays (the shifts she works). Further, she may only access information about patients on unit 2 West (the location she works) (Rinehart-Thompson 2011).

In addition to controlling how individuals access ePHI, controls can be implemented to determine how the information can be used. For example, a system may be set up to allow an individual to do one or more of the following regarding ePHI: read or view; write or create; edit; execute; append; and print.

Maintenance Records (45 CFR 164.310(a)(2)(iv))

The fourth and final implementation specification under the safeguard standard of facility access controls is maintenance records (addressable). It states that policies and procedures should be in place to ensure repairs and modifications are documented if they relate to physical areas of a facility that deal with security. Examples include repairing computer hardware; repairing or changing locks; installing new walls or doors; installing new security devices; and making routine maintenance checks. In particular, door locks may need to be rekeyed or a combination code may need to be changed if a workforce member has been terminated. Documentation in a small organization may be as simple as a notebook logging the maintenance (date, time, reason, and responsible person). In a large organization, the log may need to be maintained in a database and documented more fully (HHS 2007b).

Workstation Use (45 CFR 164.310(b))

A **workstation** is an electronic computing device and electronic media stored in the immediate vicinity. Workstations can include desktop computers, laptop computers, and other devices with similar functions (45 CFR 164.304). Workstation use (no implementation specifications) requires descriptions of what tasks may be performed at each workstation, how they may be performed, and the physical characteristics of areas surrounding workstations with access to ePHI. Threats resulting from inappropriate use include computer viruses, confidentiality breaches, and compromises to data integrity. Restrictions on workstation use extend to satellite offices and facilities, as well as remote workforce members who perform tasks at home or in other remote locations. Policies and procedures should address items such as which workstations are impacted by the rule (that is, those that access ePHI) and scheduled updates of antivirus software (HHS 2007b).

Workstation Security (45 CFR 164.310(c))

Workstation security (no implementation specifications) requires that methods be developed to protect workstations that access ePHI and restrict access to authorized users only. Workstations where ePHI is accessed may be situated in secure locations where only authorized workforce members are located or that are always monitored. The general public and passersby should not be able to view ePHI at workstations. This can be accomplished in different ways. For example, computer monitors should be turned away from public access areas, such as waiting areas. They should also be turned away from areas where coworkers without a need to access or know the information may be located (for example, hallways). Devices and software settings can also inhibit inappropriate access. For example, privacy shields can be placed over monitors to make it more difficult for passersby to read what is on them. Computers may also be programmed so monitors revert to screensaver mode after a certain period of time, which protects PHI when individuals assigned to workstations are away from the area for an extended period. Workforce members may be required to log off when their workstations will be unattended for a period of time. Computers may also be programmed to require a password to turn off the screen saver (HHS 2007b). Although the Security Rule applies only to ePHI, policies and procedures should protect both electronic and paper PHI.

Device and Media Controls (45 CFR 164.310(d)(1))

Device and media controls (four implementation specifications, two required and two addressable) require organizations to implement policies and procedures addressing the receipt and removal of hardware and electronic media that contain ePHI and move within an organization. In other words, policies and procedures must address ePHI that comes into (that is, is received) and leaves (that is, is removed from) an organization as well as ePHI within the organization. There are many types of electronic media to be tracked, including hard drives and media that can be removed and transported. Examples are magnetic tapes, magnetic or optical tapes or disks, and digital memory cards or USB flash drives. A comprehensive inventory and tracking plan must be developed with the ultimate goal of protecting ePHI (HHS 2007b).

Although the greatest risk appears to be inappropriate use (within a facility) and disclosure (leaving a facility), organizations need to closely control electronic media that comes in as well. For example, employees may bring USB drives intended for personal use into the workplace. If these devices are not closely controlled and not all media can be accounted for, an organization's inventory becomes less effective and the protection of devices and ePHI is diminished (HHS 2007b). Organizations must ask themselves whether their policies and procedures identify all types of approved and unapproved hardware and electronic media, all of which must be tracked, and whether all identified categories are being tracked thoroughly.

One of the biggest risk areas is the control of portable devices that contain ePHI. This area is particularly important because their use is growing and the likelihood of losing portable devices either accidentally or as the result of malicious acts is great. Portable devices include laptop and notebook computers, smart phones, CDs, personal digital assistants, USB drives, and handheld dictation devices. Data from the United States Department of Health and Human Services (HHS) shows that laptop theft is the most frequent cause of health information breaches, affecting 500 or more people (HHS 2012).

Disposal (45 CFR 164.310(d)(2)(i))

The first implementation specification, disposal, (required) states that policies and procedures are to be implemented to address the final disposition of ePHI, including the hardware or electronic media on which it is stored.

Media disposal can be internal or external. Internal disposal means that it is carried out by members of the organization's workforce. External disposal, to an outsourced vendor, means that the vendor is a HIPAA business associate because it is using PHI (by disposing of it) on behalf of the covered entity. Creation of a business associate agreement is therefore necessary. The business associate must comply with HIPAA requirements, including breach notification (Rinehart-Thompson 2011).

Erasing or deleting a file does not sufficiently remove ePHI. Although this function (for example, deleting a file name) will remove the pathway that leads to data, the data still exists and can be located by those with the technical know-how to do so. Policies and procedures must verify that ePHI has actually been deleted, documenting that verification, and ensure that the policies and procedures are followed. Just as an organization must realize that erasing or deleting a file does not actually remove it, the organization must also recognize that ePHI may be redundant (that is, exist in more than one location due to data backup procedures). Disposing of ePHI from one location does not necessarily remove it from the organization entirely (Rinehart-Thompson 2011).

Methods for actually destroying electronic data include degaussing, where ePHI is disrupted or actually erased through exposure to a strong magnetic field; clearing, where products overwrite the ePHI with nonsensitive data; and physical destruction or damage of electronic media prior to disposal. Destruction of electronic media includes disintegration, pulverizing, melting, incinerating, or shredding (Rinehart-Thompson 2011). Policies and procedures should specify the way(s) that ePHI, or the media it is stored on, is made unusable or inaccessible.

Whether data or electronic media is destroyed internally or the procedure is contracted to an outside organization, the destruction must be documented. A contract with an outside organization must establish the method of destruction, how the information will be protected against a breach, and how long the contractor will hold the information before it destroys it. For both internal and external destruction, a certificate or other document of destruction must verify what records were destroyed (for PHI, by individual name or identifying number); when and how they were destroyed; a statement that the destruction was in the normal course of business; and the signatures of responsible individuals and witnesses (Brodnik et al. 2012).

Media Reuse (45 CFR 164.310(d)(2)(ii))

The second implementation specification, media reuse (required), states that procedures must address the removal of ePHI from media before the media is available for reuse.

Often, an organization may want to reuse media. The Security Rule permits reuse of electronic media, which is helpful for an organization trying to be environmentally conscious while holding down costs; however, failure to remove ePHI before reuse may lead to HIPAA violations. Reuse may be internal (for example, use of an older and slower PC by an employee after a new, faster model is purchased for a coworker) or external (for example, a PC is donated to a charity or other not-for-profit organization).

As described under the first implementation specification, because erasing or deleting a file does not sufficiently remove ePHI, policies and procedures must include a way to verify that ePHI has actually been deleted or rendered inaccessible before reuse occurs (HHS 2007b).

Accountability (45 CFR 164.310(d)(2)(iii))

The third implementation specification, accountability (addressable), states that records must be maintained that track the movement of hardware and electronic media. Names of the people responsible must also be recorded. This can be extensive as it includes portable devices (such as USB drives, CDs, DVDs, and laptop computers) and other media that ePHI is often transported on such as optical disks, digital memory cards, hard drives, and magnetic tapes or disks. All types of hardware and electronic media must be identified and tracked, and care must be taken to track multiple devices of the same type through serial numbers or other tracking mechanisms (HHS 2007b).

Data Backup and Storage (45 CFR 164.310(d)(2)(iv))

The fourth and final implementation specification, data backup and storage (addressable), states that, when needed, an exact and retrievable copy of ePHI is to be created before equipment is moved. This requirement is similar to the data backup plan implementation specification in the Administrative safeguards, so the same set of policies and procedures may address both requirements. Workforce members may be required to store files on a network, thus eliminating the need to perform hard drive back-ups. Organizations should consider identifying individuals or positions responsible for creating the retrievable, exact copy and determining when it is and is not necessary to carry out this function (HHS 2007b).

CHECK YOUR UNDERSTANDING 4.1

Instructions: Indicate whether the following statements are true or false (T or F).

1. The HIPAA Security Rule imposes physical, technical, and administrative requirements to ensure the security of ePHI.
2. Large, medium, and small covered entities must all implement the HIPAA Security Rule requirements in the same way.
3. One of the greatest risks to electronic PHI is the lack of control over portable devices.
4. Deleting a file sufficiently eliminates the existence of electronic PHI.
5. One physical safeguard standard is workstation security.

Section 3: Technical Safeguards

Technical safeguards are "the technology and the policy and procedures for its use that protect electronic protected health information and control access to it" (45 CFR 164.304).

45 CFR 164.312 lists the five technical safeguards. They are outlined in figure 4.2. Implementation specifications contained within each standard are identified as either required or addressable. Standards 2 and 4, Audit Controls and Person or Entity Authentication, do not have implementation specifications.

The Security Rule does not mandate specific technologies because many workable options are available and their costs vary considerably. An organization must decide what technologies are the most reasonable and appropriate for its particular situation.

Access Control (45 CFR 164.312(a)(1))

Access control (four implementation specifications, two required and two addressable) requires policies and procedures to limit access to ePHI to only the people or software programs that require it to do their jobs. Access is "the ability or the means necessary to read, write, modify or communicate data/information or otherwise use any system resource" (45 CFR 164.304). There are a number of ways that access control can be accomplished.

FIGURE 4.2.	Technical safeguard standards		
Standards	**Sections**	**Implementation Specifications (R) = Required, (A) = Addressable**	
Access Control	§ 164.312(a)(1)	Unique User Identification	**(R)**
		Emergency Access Procedure	**(R)**
		Automatic Logoff	**(A)**
		Encryption and Decryption	**(A)**
Audit Controls	§ 164.312(b)		
Integrity	§ 164.312(c)(1)	Mechanism to Authenticate Electronic Protected Health Information	**(A)**
Person or Entity Authentication	§ 164.312(d)		
Transmission Security	§ 164.312(e)(1)	Integrity Controls	**(A)**
		Encryption	**(A)**

Source: HHS 2007c

Access must be limited to the minimum necessary for individuals to successfully perform their jobs.

Unique User Identification (45 CFR 164.312(a)(2)(i))

The first implementation specification, unique user identification (required), states that a unique name or number is to be assigned to individuals to identify and track them. That way, an organization can hold its users accountable for functions they perform in information systems that house ePHI when the users are logged into those systems (HHS 2007c). User names or numbers should be used in tandem with passwords to further identify individuals and protect ePHI. The establishment of unique identifiers is discussed further under the technical safeguard standard of "person or entity authentication."

Emergency Access Procedure (45 CFR 164.312(a)(2)(ii))

The second implementation specification, emergency access procedure (required), states that procedures are to be established to obtain necessary ePHI during emergencies. When an emergency occurs, an individual may need to access information that would otherwise be denied because of controls that have been built into the system. Before an emergency occurs, an organization needs to determine what types of situations warrant access and create instructions for gaining access. Emergency access may be necessary when normal systems are not operable (for example, due to a disruption in electrical power). Emergency access may also be necessary when systems are operable, but an individual needs to access ePHI that they otherwise would not have access rights to at that time. **"Break the glass"** is a system capability that allows an individual who otherwise does not have access privileges to ePHI to access it through an alternative method in limited, necessary situations. For example, Ellen is a nurse who may have been assigned to a different shift, but her system access was not changed. An emergency situation might have necessitated her "breaking the glass" to access information about one of her patients. Ellen should only do this if it was absolutely necessary to access the information and her access level could not have been changed through standard methods. Policies and procedures should identify situations that warrant breaking the glass and should be written to minimize the frequency of occurrences. After an individual breaks the glass, each situation should be specifically audited for appropriateness (Rinehart-Thompson 2011).

Automatic Log-Off (45 CFR 164.312(a)(2)(iii))

The third implementation specification, automatic log-off (addressable), provides for termination of electronic sessions on workstations that access ePHI. Users should log off whenever they leave their workstations, but they can easily forget or not be able to because they are occupied with other duties. This is a problem in any area where unauthorized individuals might be able to access ePHI. For example, members of the public or other employees may be able to see private information left on computer screens in patient registration departments or nursing units. The automatic log-off feature secures ePHI by ending a computer session after a predetermined period of inactivity. This feature helps to prevent unauthorized access to ePHI when it is left unattended. Network administrators or an organization's management team may set the period of time that elapses before log-off occurs. It can be as immediate as one minute or as long as ten minutes or longer.

An alternative to an automatic log-off mechanism is activation of a password-protected screen saver. As opposed to a log-off, which takes a user out of a system, a screen saver simply makes it impossible to see the information (which is "hidden" behind the screen saver design that has been selected) until someone with the appropriate password activates the screen so it can be viewed. As an addressable implementation specification, an organization has options in determining the best way to protect unattended ePHI. In either case, the ePHI is no longer visible (HHS 2007c).

Encryption and Decryption (45 CFR 164.312(a)(2)(iv))

The fourth and final implementation specification, encryption and decryption (addressable), provides for a mechanism to encrypt and decrypt ePHI.

Encryption (scrambling or encoding of data) and **decryption** (restoration of data) are based on **cryptography**, a science that uses mathematical algorithms to change meaningful information into unintelligible data, similar to a code. This process protects data from being read while it is in transit. At its destination, data reverts back to meaningful information when an authorized user receives it. Because there is a risk that health data will be intercepted during transmission, resulting in privacy breaches, encryption is an important and powerful security mechanism. Encryption is also the desired mechanism to protect ePHI on portable devices which—because of their mobility—can be easily lost or stolen (Rinehart-Thompson 2011).

Encryption is addressed twice in the technical safeguard standards, under Access Control and Transmission Security. In each case encryption is addressable rather than required. Despite the fact that the Security Rule does not specifically require encryption, it has nonetheless become an industry expectation. Because the cost of encryption continues to decrease, it makes sense to encrypt whenever possible. Because encrypted information is considered secure, HIPAA's breach notification interim final rule exempts properly-encrypted PHI from breach notification requirements.

There are two types of encryption: asymmetric (public key infrastructure) and symmetric (private key infrastructure, or single-key encryption). The sending computer's keys encrypt the information and the recipient computer's keys decrypt or decode the information back to the original text.

Public key infrastructure (PKI) is the most common method of encryption technology. It uses two keys to encrypt, transmit, and send a message. The sending computer has a private key to code the message, and it gives a public key to the receiving computer. The receiving computer uses the public key to decode the message. The identity of the receiving computer and its relationship to the public key is confirmed by an independent certification authority (CA). A digital certificate, issued to the receiving computer, acts as a verification of authenticity.

In **private key infrastructure**, both the sending and receiving computers use software that assigns a secret code, or key. Both computers must have the same key for this technology to work. The key is used by the sending computer to code (scramble) the data. The same key is used by the receiving computer to decode (unscramble) the data. This method is not as secure because the key, which decodes the information, is transmitted with the data. An experienced computer hacker could intercept the key and use it to decode the accompanying data. Not all keys have the same level of strength and robustness. The more robust the key, the more secure the information.

With attention focused on the theft of electronic devices, especially portable devices such as laptops, a variety of encryption methods are becoming more common. **Self-encrypted hard drives** protect their own data by encrypting it through keys that reside on the drive itself. Only the correct password can unlock or decrypt the data. **Full disk encryption** signifies that all data present on the disk is encrypted.

Audit Controls (45 CFR 164.312(b))

Audit controls (no implementation specifications) require installation of hardware, software, or manual mechanisms to examine and record activity in systems containing ePHI. Audit controls occur at the back end, after activity has occurred, rather than preventatively.

One type of audit control is the **audit trail** (also known as **audit log**), a feature that records access or access attempts in a computer system. Although retrospective, it can provide valuable **metadata** (data about data) including who accessed (or attempted to access) the system; which part or parts of the system were affected; when the access occurred; what operations occurred (such as create, view, print, edit); and when data was sent and received. This metadata can be used for investigations (and potential disciplinary actions), breach notification, and other mitigation efforts (Rinehart-Thompson 2011). The Security Rule does not mandate what information must be collected in an audit report or how frequently audit reports must be generated and reviewed. **Intrusion detection systems** analyze network traffic, sending an alarm if they detect potentially inappropriate attempts to access the network or a particular account. This system cannot operate independently, but requires humans to monitor alarms and determine whether or not they are valid. An organization's characteristics, as well as findings from a risk analysis, should determine what are reasonable and appropriate audit controls (HHS 2007c).

Although the audit controls standard addresses the examination and recording of activity that is occurring or has occurred in systems containing ePHI, there are other mechanisms that can preventatively identify abnormal conditions in an electronic system. **Intrusion prevention systems** identify inappropriate traffic, blocking passage in much the same way as a firewall, which provides a security barrier between an internal trusted network and outside electronic traffic. Like the intrusion detection system, this system also requires humans to monitor alarms and determine whether or not they are valid (Rinehart-Thompson 2011).

Systems can also be set up to respond preventatively to an established threshold of **invalid log-on attempts** (use of an incorrect user name or password) to a particular account. After the established number of attempts is reached, additional attempts are prohibited through an **account lockout**. The account lockout may continue for a specified period of time that has been programmed into the system, or until the network administrator manually unlocks it (Rinehart-Thompson 2011).

Integrity (45 CFR 164.312(c)(1))

Integrity (one implementation specification, which is addressable) requires policies and procedures that protect ePHI from being altered or destroyed in an unauthorized manner.

Integrity refers to data that has maintained its structure and attributes. Accuracy and completeness are important aspects of data integrity, as are the lack of unauthorized modification or corruption (AHIMA 2012). If health information's integrity is compromised, there are many potential consequences. However, the greatest one is the threat to patient safety due to incorrect or omitted information. There are a number of reasons that unauthorized alteration or destruction might occur. Electronic media failures, human error, or malicious human acts can all affect the integrity of ePHI. Policies and procedures must be written to respond to any of these causes.

Mechanism to Authenticate Electronic Protected Health Information (45 CFR 164.312(c)(2))

This implementation specification (addressable) provides for electronic mechanisms to corroborate that ePHI has not been altered or destroyed in an unauthorized manner. An audit trail, which provides metadata, can be a powerful tool to detect unauthorized activities. However, it requires personnel to follow up on the data that is generated. Organizations must first identify the risk to ePHI integrity through a risk analysis. Based on this information, security measures must be identified to reduce those risks. Finally, those security measures must be put into action (HHS 2007c).

Person or Entity Authentication (45 CFR 164.312(d))

Person authentication or **entity authentication** (no implementation specifications) requires procedures to prevent unauthorized users from accessing ePHI by verifying that a person is who he says he is. This standard operates in conjunction with the Access Control standard's implementation specification of unique user identification.

Authentication allows an individual to access a system only after information that corroborates the identity of who the individual claims to be has been provided. Using predetermined criteria to verify that a user is who he says he is, a person may authenticate himself by entering information that matches what has been stored in the system. A person may authenticate himself in one of three ways (or a combination thereof): what the user knows; what the user has; and what the user is. Use of any one of the three mechanisms is **single-factor authentication**, whereas a combination of two of the mechanisms is two-factor authentication. **Two-factor authentication** provides greater security than one-factor authentication.

"What the user knows" (that is, combining user names and passwords) is generally considered the least secure. The user name (also referred to as a user ID or log-on ID) is a unique identifier used to track an individual's activity in a system. Containing letters of the alphabet, numbers, or a combination of both, it is generally known by others and fairly easy to figure out (for example, jdoe for Jane Doe). Because it can be easily figured out, it must be used in conjunction with a password to authenticate a user's identity. Passwords are meant to be secret, and thus known only by the user. Computer systems often create requirements for passwords, forcing users to create ones that the system's administrators consider robust enough for adequate security (Rinehart-Thompson 2011). Passwords are the most common authentication mechanism, but other methods should be explored as well due to the risk of passwords being posted, lost, stolen, or decoded. Figure 4.3 provides tips for more secure passwords.

FIGURE 4.3.	Tips for secure passwords

- Use and intersperse a combination of numbers, alphabetic characters, and symbols (for example, #, $, %)
- Use both upper-case and lower-case letters, inserting capitals in unexpected places (for example, in the middle of the password)
- Use a sufficient number of characters (eight characters is better than six characters)
- Create a password that is meaningful so the user can recall it, but others cannot
- Create a password that appears to be random to others
- Regularly change or update passwords (the system may automatically require this)
- Do not use common words or phrases, particularly if they can be linked to the person who created them (for example, a family member's name or birth month)
- Do not use a date that is known to be associated with the user (for example, birthdate or anniversary)
- Do not use nouns or proper names (such as nicknames, places, newsworthy terms, sports teams, celebrities)
- Do not use words that appear in a dictionary (either English or another language)
- Do not use a password that is the same as or similar to the user's actual name, the username, or e-mail address
- Do not select a password that is similar to the previous password
- Do not store passwords where they can be accessed by others

Source: Cazier and Medlin 2006

"What the user has" is the second authentication method. It relies on something the user has in his or her possession (a token) such as a key card. Alone (single-factor authentication) it provides insufficient security because of how easily it can be lost, stolen, or misplaced. It should be combined with a password or personal identification number (PIN) for enhanced two-factor authentication (Rinehart-Thompson 2011).

"What the user is," the third authentication method, uses biometric identifiers to grant access to a system. The system analyzes biological data such as fingerprints, palm vein scans, face prints, retinal scans, and full-body scans. A reader or scanning device uses software to convert the scanned information into a digital format. A database that stores the biometric data then compares it to grant access (Rinehart-Thompson 2011). This is the most secure method, but some individuals may resist having their biological data collected and stored (particularly by their employer), viewing it as an invasion of their personal privacy.

In addition to authentication an organization can control individuals' ability to access ePHI: user-based, role-based, and context-based access. These were discussed in section 2: Physical Safeguards.

Transmission Security (45 CFR 164.312(e)(1))

Transmission security (two implementation specifications, both addressable) provides for measures to be taken that protect ePHI against unauthorized access when it is being transmitted via an electronic communications network. Organizations must first identify how ePHI is being transmitted (for example, e-mail, via the Internet, private networks) in order to determine appropriate ways to protect it (HHS 2007c). Once this is done, options can be explored. These include the types of encryption discussed earlier in the chapter. As the costs associated with encryption data continue to decrease, concerns about encryption being cost-prohibitive should also diminish.

Integrity Controls (45 CFR 164.312(e)(2)(i))

The first implementation specification, integrity controls (addressable), states that security measures should be implemented so electronically transmitted ePHI will not be improperly modified without detection. This implementation specification relates to the integrity standard except that the context of integrity controls is specifically data transmission.

Different types of integrity control mechanisms may provide security when data are transmitted. A **firewall** is a buffer between an organization's internal (trusted) network and the Internet, which is considered an untrusted network. The firewall evaluates information that enters and exits the internal network. Based on predetermined system rules, information may be prevented from either entering or exiting. Further, users in the internal network may be prevented from accessing information on the Internet and external users may be prevented from accessing the internal network. A firewall may be able to stop some viruses, but not others. **Antivirus software packages** may be installed to check for, detect, and block viruses that have been introduced into a system. Because new viruses are constantly being created, an organization's catalog of viruses must be continuously updated and the organization's computers must be routinely scanned for viruses (Rinehart-Thompson 2011).

Encryption (45 CFR 164.312(e)(2)(ii))

The second and final implementation specification, encryption (addressable), states that mechanisms to encrypt ePHI should be implemented whenever the organization finds it appropriate to do so. Encryption was discussed as one of the addressable implementation specifications of the Access Control standard. Here, it relates specifically to the transmission of data. Encryption for transmitting ePHI over the Internet should be given the highest priority due to the significant risk it presents. However, the Security Rule allows flexibility in determining what methods, when, and with whom encryption will be used. Organizations should discuss encryption methods with its vendors, IT staff, and other entities with which it exchanges ePHI (HHS 2007c).

CHECK YOUR UNDERSTANDING 4.2

Instructions: Indicate whether the following statements are true or false (T or F).

1. Decryption is the restoration of scrambled or coded data.
2. Private key infrastructure is a less secure method of encryption because the key that decodes the information is transmitted with the data.
3. An intrusion detection system can be set up to operate automatically without human monitoring.
4. An individual's user name should be the same as his or her password.
5. A firewall protects against the unauthorized transmission of ePHI between two computers within an internal network.

Section 4: Administrative Safeguards

Administrative safeguards are "administrative actions, and policies and procedures, to manage the selection, development, implementation, and maintenance of security measures to protect electronic protected health information and to manage the conduct of the covered entity's workforce in relation to the protection of that information" (45 CFR 164.304). Over half of HIPAA's security requirements are administrative safeguards. The HIPAA Security Rule's administrative safeguards are the foundation of an organization's security program.

The nine administrative safeguards are listed in 45 CFR 164.308. They are outlined in figure 4.4. Implementation specifications contained within each standard are identified as either required or addressable. Standards 2 and 8, Assigned Security Responsibility and Evaluation, do not have implementation specifications.

FIGURE 4.4.	Administrative safeguard standards		
Standards	**Sections**	**Implementation Specifications (R) = Required, (A) = Addressable**	
Security Management Process	§ 164.308(a)(1)	Risk Analysis	**(R)**
		Risk Management	**(R)**
		Sanction Policy	**(R)**
		Information System Activity Review	**(R)**
Assigned Security Responsibility	§ 164.308(a)(2)		
Workforce Security	§ 164.308(a)(3)	Authorization and/or Supervision	**(A)**
		Workforce Clearance Procedure	**(A)**
		Termination Procedures	**(A)**

(Continued on next page)

FIGURE 4.4.	(Continued)		
Standards	**Sections**	**Implementation Specifications** **(R) = Required, (A) = Addressable**	
Information Access Management	§ 164.308(a)(4)	Isolating Health Care Clearinghouse Functions	**(R)**
		Access Authorization	**(A)**
		Access Establishment and Modification	**(A)**
Security Awareness and Training	§ 164.308(a)(5)	Security Reminders	**(A)**
		Protection from Malicious Software	**(A)**
		Log-in Monitoring	**(A)**
		Password Management	**(A)**
Security Incident Procedures	§ 164.308(a)(6)	Response and Reporting	**(R)**
Contingency Plan	§ 164.308(a)(7)	Data Backup Plan	**(R)**
		Disaster Recovery Plan	**(R)**
		Emergency Mode Operation Plan	**(R)**
		Testing and Revision Procedures	**(A)**
		Applications and Data Criticality Analysis	**(A)**
Evaluation	§ 164.308(a)(8)		
Business Associate Contracts and Other Arrangements	§ 164.308(b)(1)	Written Contract or Other Arrangement	**(R)**

Source: HHS 2007a

Security Management Process (45 CFR 164.308(a)(1))

Security management process (four implementation specifications, all required) requires the implementation of policies and procedures to prevent, detect, contain, and correct security violations. It highlights the importance of the first two implementation specifications, risk analysis and risk management, and provides for appropriate sanctions for security violations. This standard and its implementation specifications form the foundation of an organization's security activities (HHS 2007a).

Risk Analysis (45 CFR 164.308(a)(1)(ii)(A))

The first implementation specification, risk analysis (required), states that organizations are to conduct an accurate and thorough assessment of potential risks and vulnerabilities that will affect the confidentiality, integrity, and availability of ePHI. An assessment should look at both the likelihood (probability) of the risk actually occurring, as well as the magnitude of the occurrence.

To complete an analysis, an organization should look at how ePHI flows throughout the organization (including ePHI that is received, created, maintained, and transmitted). Both internal sources of ePHI (such as portable devices) and external sources of ePHI (such as that created by vendors or consultants) should be considered, as should human and natural threats to ePHI (HHS 2007a).

Risk Management (45 CFR 164.308(a)(1)(ii)(B))

The second implementation specification, risk management (required), states that security measures should be implemented that are sufficient to reduce risks and vulnerabilities to a level that is reasonable and appropriate for complying with the Security Rule's general requirements for protecting ePHI. In other words, an organization must decide how it will address security risks and vulnerabilities. The risk management concept is not unique to ePHI security. **Risk management** applies to all aspects of an organization's operations and focuses on identifying, evaluating and controlling risks that can expose the organization to financial liability (AHIMA 2012). As with any area that can result in financial liability, an organization should look at its security measures that are already in place and ask itself whether they are adequate or whether gaps still exist. Further, a risk management program will not be effective without commitment from those in top leadership positions. Executive leaders should be involved in the development and support of security measures. Finally, a knowledgeable workforce is critical. The organization must communicate to all workforce members about security measures (HHS 2007a). As described in chapter 2, workforce members include paid employees; employees of outsourced vendors who work routinely on the premises; unpaid volunteers, trainees, and student interns; and anyone working under the covered entity's or business associate's direct control.

Sanction Policy (45 CFR 164.308(a)(1)(ii)(C))

The third implementation specification, sanction policy (required), states that covered entities are to appropriately sanction workforce members who do not comply with the organization's security policies and procedures. Employees and prospective employees should sign statements agreeing to abide by the organization's policies and procedures, and acknowledging that violation may lead to disciplinary action, up to termination depending on the severity of the infraction (HHS 2007a). Not all instances of noncompliance warrant termination. An organization's human resources department must have thorough policies and procedures in place to identify the appropriate disciplinary action for various types of infractions. While intentional breaches (for example, snooping in the health record of a celebrity or coworker) may warrant termination, policies may provide for lesser actions such as verbal or written reprimands, or paid or unpaid suspensions, for less egregious violations. These may include posting or sharing passwords, or routinely failing to log out when leaving one's workstation.

Information System Activity Review (45 CFR 164.308(a)(1)(ii)(D))

The fourth and final implementation specification, information system activity review (required), states that records of information systems, such as audit logs, access reports, and security incident tracking reports, are to be reviewed regularly. This enables the inappropriate use or detection of ePHI to be detected. An organization should be aware of the types of reports its information system can generate, and use them as fully as possible according to what is appropriate for that organization's characteristics and risk factors (HHS 2007a).

Assigned Security Responsibility (45 CFR 164.308(a)(2))

Assigned security responsibility (no implementation specifications) requires that organizations identify the individual responsible for overseeing the development and implementation of the organization's security policies and procedures. This requirement is a corollary to the Privacy Rule's requirement that a privacy officer also be designated. The privacy officer and security officer may be (but is not required to be) the same person. Also, individuals may be assigned specific security tasks although one person is given overall responsibility (HHS 2007a).

Workforce Security (45 CFR 164.308(a)(3))

Workforce security (three implementation specifications, all addressable) requires policies and procedures that ensure members of the workforce have access to ePHI appropriate for their jobs, and that also prevent unauthorized access to ePHI. For each person who is identified as needing access to ePHI, the organization must identify what is needed (that is, the minimum necessary) and when it is needed, and control access to it (HHS 2007a). An organization must decide whether it will implement UBAC, RBAC, or CBAC, all discussed previously in this chapter. The level of access given to individuals, by any of these methods, must be routinely reviewed and updated.

Authorization and/or Supervision (45 CFR 164.308(a)(3)(ii)(A))

The first implementation specification, authorization and/or supervision (addressable), states that procedures are to be implemented for the authorization and/or supervision of workforce members working with ePHI or in locations where ePHI might be accessed. This implementation specification is designed to provide checks and balances for appropriate access (which, for some workforce members, may be no access). For example, this process will determine whether a particular employee has the right to perform a certain activity (such as, reading, editing, printing, or running a program). The size of the organization will affect this provision. For instance, dental offices are often small with office and clinical staff supporting only one or two dentists. In a small office such as this, it is unlikely that each staff member will have just one role. Instead, they will most likely be cross-trained on a number of functions. As a result, each staff member may need to access all ePHI in the system. On the other hand, workforce members in a large hospital will have more specialized tasks. Organizations should have detailed job descriptions that will elicit the access rights of each workforce member; determine who has authority to grant access rights; and review policies and procedures that are already in place (HHS 2007a).

Workforce Clearance Procedure (45 CFR 164.308(a)(3)(ii)(B))

The second implementation specification, workforce clearance procedure (addressable), states that procedures should "determine that the access of a workforce member to ePHI is appropriate" (45 CFR 164.308(a)(3)(ii)(b)). In other words, procedures must be in place to "clear" a workforce member for a certain level of access. This screening may occur as part of the authorization or supervision procedure just described. In larger organizations, it will often involve approval by a workforce member's manager. In smaller organizations, all approvals may be channeled through one person who serves as the security officer. These procedures must be applied consistently throughout the organization.

Termination Procedures (45 CFR 164.308(a)(3)(ii)(C))

The third and final implementation specification, termination procedures (addressable), states that procedures must be in place to terminate access to ePHI when a workforce member's employment or relationship with the organization ends or if the workforce clearance procedure, discussed in the previous section, requires termination of access privileges. The procedure applies regardless of whether the individual leaves the organization voluntarily or involuntarily. The same procedure used for termination should also be used when a workforce member's access level changes (to either more or less access) due to a job description change. Responsibility for carrying out this task should be assigned to ensure it is completed. Further, terminations and job description changes must be communicated in a timely manner so the procedures can be followed immediately (HHS 2007a).

Information Access Management (45 CFR 164.308(a)(4))

Information access management (three implementation specifications, one required and two addressable) requires organizations to implement procedures authorizing access to ePHI consistent with the Privacy Rule. In particular, organizations must ensure compliance with the minimum necessary requirements.

Isolating Healthcare Clearinghouse Functions (45 CFR 164.308(a)(4)(ii)(A))

The first implementation specification, isolating healthcare clearinghouse functions (required), states that a healthcare clearinghouse that is part of a larger organization "must implement policies and procedures that protect the ePHI of the clearinghouse from unauthorized access by the larger organization" (45 CFR 164.308(a)(4)(ii)(A)). Organizations with a healthcare clearinghouse as one of its functions must review its technical safeguards to determine whether specific procedures are needed to separate ePHI in the clearinghouse's information systems from the larger organization (HHS 2007a).

Access Authorization (45 CFR 164.308(a)(4)(ii)(B))

The second implementation specification, access authorization (addressable), states that policies and procedures should be implemented—if reasonable and appropriate—"for granting access to ePHI" (45 CFR 164.308(a)(4)(ii)(B)). Examples of avenues for accessing ePHI include workstations and software programs. The policies and procedures must identify who is given authority to grant access privileges and what process those individuals must follow. Authorization should be documented, and authorization and clearance procedures should be followed. Technical processes, such as assigning user names, should be followed as well (HHS 2007a).

Access Establishment and Modification (45 CFR 164.308(a)(4)(ii)(C))

The third and final implementation specification, access establishment and modification (addressable), states that policies and procedures are to be implemented that, "based upon the entity's access authorization policies, establish, document, review, and modify a user's right of access to a workstation, transaction, program, or process" (45 CFR 164.308(a)(4)(ii)(C)). This requires the management of access privileges. This responsibility may be given to individuals who also have authority for terminating access privileges. As part of this implementation specification, procedures should provide for a periodic review of workforce members' actual access and levels of access to make sure they are consistent with what they are authorized to access.

Security Awareness and Training (45 CFR 164.308(a)(5))

Security awareness and training (four implementation specifications, all addressable) require a "security awareness and training program for all members of its workforce (including management)" (45 CFR 164.308(a)(5)(i)). This standard emphasizes that no safeguard will completely protect ePHI if the workforce is not aware of its responsibilities. Humans can be the most significant element in weak information security, so workforce awareness and behaviors must be addressed through awareness and training. It may be tailored to meet the organization's needs, but it must be provided for both new and existing workforce members. Additionally, training updates should be provided. Training should include changes to the Security Rule; policies and procedures (and updates when they occur); new or upgraded hardware and software; and new technologies that enhance security (HHS 2007a).

Security Reminders (45 CFR 164.308(a)(5)(ii)(A))

The first implementation specification, security reminders (addressable), states that periodic security updates must be provided. Notification can occur through electronic or printed materials, as part of meeting agendas, or during trainings. For example, workforce members may be reminded, through any of these avenues, to log out of the system when they leave their workstations or to change their passwords every 90 days (this is particularly necessary if the system does not lock out individuals for failure to update their passwords). Routine retraining sessions may also be scheduled at predetermined intervals (for example, annually). It is important to continually assess whether the reminders are providing sufficient communication to the workforce (HHS 2007a).

Protection from Malicious Software (45 CFR 164.308(a)(5)(ii)(B))

The second implementation specification, protection from malicious software (addressable), states that there are to be "procedures for guarding against, detecting, and reporting malicious software" where reasonable and appropriate (45 CFR 164.308(a)(5)(ii)(B)). Malicious software is any unauthorized program that can infiltrate an information system, causing harm to the system or its data or requiring repairs that cost the organization in terms of time and money. Users are most familiar with viruses, Trojan horses, or worms. Workforce training, the previous implementation specification discussed, is an important part of protecting information systems because items such as e-mail attachments, downloadable programs from the Internet, and documents brought into the organization on portable devices such as USB drives may introduce malicious software. The workforce can be instrumental in either protecting the information system or introducing new risks (HHS 2007a).

Log-In Monitoring (45 CFR 164.308(a)(5)(ii)(C))

The third implementation specification, log-in monitoring (addressable), states that procedures should be in place to monitor log-in attempts and report questionable activity. Monitoring can include tracking attempts to access a system through multiple combinations of user names and passwords. Monitoring may occur manually, or through the creation of audit trails (audit logs). As noted previously, audit trails can be generated automatically; however, the results must be monitored by individuals. Particularly where additional investigation is needed, this may require a significant expenditure of human resources. Systems might also automatically require a period of inactivity or a password to be reset after a particular number of suspicious attempts. Workforce members should be trained on logging into systems and managing their passwords (HHS 2007a).

Password Management (45 CFR 164.308(a)(5)(ii)(D))

The fourth and final implementation specification, password management (addressable), states that procedures should be established "for creating, changing, and safeguarding passwords" (45 CFR 164.308(a)(5)(ii)(D)). Workforce members must be made aware of guidelines for password creation and password change cycles. Policies should exist to prohibit password sharing and advise workforce members to memorize their passwords rather than writing them down and making them visible to others (HHS 2007a).

Security Incident Procedures (45 CFR 164.308(a)(6))

Security incident procedures (one implementation specification, required) provide for policies and procedures for reporting and responding to security incidents. A security incident is when someone makes an unauthorized attempt (either successfully or unsuccessfully) to access, use, disclose, modify or destroy information, or to interfere with the operation of an information system. For example, a procedure should be in place to respond to multiple unsuccessful log-in attempts to a user's account (the procedure should specify the number of attempts that the organization deems suspicious enough to trigger a response). When an individual needs to "break the glass" (described earlier in the chapter), the situation should be responded to per a written procedure. Although the other standards in the Security Rule are designed to reduce the number of security incidents, they will still occur (HHS 2007a).

Response and Reporting (45 CFR 164.308(a)(6)(ii))

The implementation specification of response and reporting (required), states that suspected and known security incidents must be identified and responded to. The incident must be reported and documented. Appropriate responses to security incidents must be communicated to workforce members and may include preserving evidence, mitigating the harmful effects to the extent it is practical to do so, knowing who to report the incident to, documenting the incident, and evaluating the incident as part of the overall risk management process. Possible incidents include inappropriate access and use of passwords; corrupted backup tapes; virus attacks; physical break-ins with subsequent ePHI theft; failure to terminate accounts of former workforce members (with subsequent unauthorized use); and providing media containing ePHI to an unauthorized user (HHS 2007a).

Contingency Plan (45 CFR 164.308(a)(7))

Contingency plan (five implementation specifications, three required and two address-able) requires an organization to develop and implement policies and procedures for responding to an emergency or occurrence (such as a flood, tornado, or fire) that damages equipment or systems containing ePHI such that information is not available to caregivers when and where it is needed. The plan includes recovering access to ePHI (HHS 2007a).

Data Backup Plan (45 CFR 164.308(a)(7)(ii)(A))

The first implementation specification, data backup plan (required), states that procedures are to be implemented to "create and maintain retrievable, exact copies of ePHI" (HHS 2007a). This ensures backup procedures as part of an organization's business practices. Procedures should detail what ePHI is to be backed up, including all important ePHI source systems (such as accounting, electronic health records, case management information, diagnostic images and electronic test results, and other electronic documents). Alternative backup methods should be considered, as well as the frequency of backups and the storage of backup media in a safe and secure location (HHS 2007a).

Disaster Recovery Plan (45 CFR 164.308(a)(7)(ii)(B))

The second implementation specification, disaster recovery plan (required), states that procedures should be in place to restore lost data. This may be included in an organization's disaster plan, but this must be determined. The plan must also determine what data are to be restored and whether a copy of the disaster plan is readily accessible at multiple locations (HHS 2007a).

Emergency Mode Operation Plan (45 CFR 164.308(a)(7)(ii)(C))

The third implementation specification, emergency mode operation plan (required), states that procedures should be in place to allow "continuation of critical business processes for protection of the security of ePHI while operating in emergency mode" (45 CFR 164.308(a)(7)(ii)(C)). An emergency mode of operations is required in cases such as a technical failure of the system or a power outage. This involves balancing the need to access data with the need to protect it. The emergency mode plan must also consider alternative security measures, potential manual procedures, and contact information of those who must be notified (HHS 2007a).

Testing and Revision Procedures (45 CFR 164.308(a)(7)(ii)(D))

The fourth implementation specification, testing and revision procedures (address-able), provides for "procedures for periodic testing and revision of contingency plans" (45 CFR 164.308(a)(7)(ii)(D)). This applies to all plans with implementation specifications under the contingency plan standard (data backup plan, disaster recovery plan, and emergency mode operation plan). Options for testing include hypotheticals, scenario-based walk-throughs and live tests. These processes (and the results of each test) are to be documented and responsible persons identified (HHS 2007a).

Applications and Data Criticality Analysis (45 CFR 164.308(a)(7)(ii)(E))

The fifth and final implementation specification, applications and data criticality analysis (addressable), provides that an organization is to "assess the relative criticality of specific applications and data in support of other contingency plan components" (45 CFR 164.308(a)(7)(ii)(E)). It includes the identification of software applications that store, maintain, or transmit ePHI, determining which are the most important for patient care or other business operations. Based on this prioritization, decisions will be made about data backup, disaster recovery, and emergency operations plans. The priority list will be used to decide what data are restored first and what data has to be available at all times (HHS 2007a). This process will be followed organization-wide; however, the health information department will follow a similar process specific to its own operations. For example, it may determine that patient identification (that is, the master patient index) is a priority and, consequently, this data will be restored first and thereafter be continually available.

Evaluation (45 CFR 164.308(a)(8))

Evaluation (no implementation specifications) requires an organization to implement continuous monitoring and evaluation. This is required because it is important for an organization to know whether its security plans actually protect ePHI adequately. The standard requires a "periodic technical and a nontechnical evaluation, based initially upon the standards implemented under this rule and subsequently, in response to environmental or operations changes" (45 CFR164.308(a)(8)). Organizations must determine the frequency of evaluations and whether special evaluations should be conducted if security incidents occur. Documentation of evaluations must also be completed (HHS 2007a). The evaluation process can be incorporated into an organization's quality improvement initiatives.

Business Associate Contracts and Other Arrangements (45 CFR 164.308(b)(1))

Business associate contracts and other arrangements (one implementation specification, required) requires that contracts between a covered entity and its business associates provide satisfactory assurance that appropriate safeguards will be applied to protect ePHI created, received, maintained, or transmitted on behalf of the covered entity. Business associates frequently handle ePHI while working to carry on the business of the covered entities with which they have relationships. This standard highlights the important role of business associates in safeguarding ePHI. There are limited exceptions to this standard for the transmission of ePHI by a covered entity to a healthcare provider for treatment; and transmissions involving health plans and government programs.

Written Contract or Other Arrangement (45 CFR 164.308(b)(4))

The implementation specification of written contract or other arrangement (required) states the satisfactory assurances that business associates will protect ePHI must be documented via a written contract or other acceptable arrangement. All business associates must be identified, with contracts including provisions for ePHI. If possible, existing business associate contracts can be modified to include both Privacy Rule and Security Rule requirements.

Section 5: Organizational Requirements

45 CFR 164.314 lists the two organizational requirement standards in the HIPAA Security Rule. They are outlined in figure 4.5. The implementation specifications contained within each standard are required.

Business Associate Contracts or Other Arrangements (45 CFR 164.314(a)(1))

Business associate contracts or other arrangements (two implementation specifications, both required) state that a business associate agreement or other type of arrangement must be in place between a covered entity and its business associates that will be accessing the covered entity's ePHI. The language used can vary as long as it still meets the requirements. Additionally, the requirements of the contract or arrangement must be enforced; otherwise, this standard is not met. For example, if a business associate commits a material breach or violation of the contract or agreement and the covered entity takes no action to respond to it, the standard is violated (HHS 2007d).

Business Associate Contracts (45 CFR 164.314(a)(2)(i))

The first implementation specification, business associate contracts (required), states that a contract between a covered entity and its business associate must provide that the business associate will do the following:

- "Implement administrative, physical, and technical safeguards that reasonably and appropriately protect the confidentiality, integrity, and availability of the ePHI that it creates, receives, maintains, or transmits on behalf of the covered entity;
- Ensure that any agent, including a subcontractor, to whom it provides such information agrees to implement reasonable and appropriate safeguards to protect it;
- Report to the covered entity any security incident of which it becomes aware;
- Authorize termination of the contract by the covered entity, if the covered entity determines that the business associate has violated a material term of the contract." (45 CFR 164.314(a)(2)(i))

Business associate agreements must comply with the HIPAA Privacy and Security Rules (the latter being applicable if business associates create, receive, maintain, or transmit ePHI) (HHS 2007d). Business associate agreements must comply with the HITECH requirements.

FIGURE 4.5.	Organizational requirements		
Standards	Sections	Implementation Specifications (R) = Required, (A) = Addressable	
Business Associate Contracts or Other Arrangements	§ 164.314(a)(1)	Business Associate Contracts	(R)
		Other Arrangements	(R)
Requirements for Group Health Plans	§ 164.314(b)(1)	Implementation Specifications	(R)

Source: HHS 2007d

Other Arrangements (45 CFR 164.314(a)(2)(ii))

The second and final implementation specification, other arrangements (required), states that when a covered entity and its business associate are both government organizations, the covered entity can comply with the Security Rule (1) via a memorandum of understanding (MOU) that meets the Security Rule's business associate agreement requirements; or (2) if other law, including regulations adopted by the covered entity or the business associate, contains requirements that accomplish the business associate agreement objectives. The portion of the agreement that permits a covered entity to terminate the agreement may be omitted if statutory obligations do not permit its inclusion (HHS 2007d). This section has narrow application because, in the majority of situations, both a covered entity and its business associate are not government organizations. One example where this provision could apply is if a state department of mental health or developmental disabilities (government agencies) uses another government agency to process claims for services provided.

Group Health Plans (45 CFR 164.314(b)(1))

The group health plans standard (one implementation specification, required) states that "a group health plan must ensure that its plan documents provide that the plan sponsor will reasonably and appropriately safeguard ePHI created, received, maintained, or transmitted to or by the plan sponsor on behalf of the group health plan" (45 CFR 164.314(b)(1)). The exception is when the only ePHI disclosed to a plan sponsor is done so pursuant to Privacy Rule permitted disclosures (summary information to the plan sponsor; participation or enrollment in the group health plan; or pursuant to an authorization or one of the Privacy Rule's authorization exceptions) (HHS 2007d).

Implementation Specifications (45 CFR 164.314(b)(2))

The implementation specification, the only one in the rule titled "implementation specifications" (required), states that the plan documents of the group health plan must incorporate provisions that require the plan sponsor to

- "Implement administrative, physical, and technical safeguards that reasonably and appropriately protect the confidentiality, integrity and availability of the ePHI that it creates, receives, maintains, or transmits on behalf of the group health plan";
- Ensure that the adequate separation required by 164.504(f)(2)(iii) of the Privacy Rule is supported by reasonable and appropriate security measures;

- Ensure that any agent, including a subcontractor, to whom it provides this information agrees to implement reasonable and appropriate security mechanisms to protect the information; and
- Report to the group health plan any security incident of which it becomes aware" (45 CFR 164.314(b)(2))

If a group health plan's plan sponsor has access to ePHI beyond summary and enrollment information or that authorized by section 164.508 of the Privacy Rule (pertaining to authorizations), language in the plan documents must be similar to language that the Privacy Rule already requires (HHS 2007d).

Section 6: Policies and Procedures and Documentation

45 CFR 164.316 lists the policies and procedures and documentation standards in the HIPAA Security Rule. They are outlined in figure 4.6. There are no implementation specifications for policies and procedures. The implementation specifications for documentation are all required.

Policies and Procedures (45 CFR 164.316(a))

The policies and procedures standard (no implementation specifications) lists the policy and procedure requirements. It states that reasonable and appropriate policies and procedures are to be implemented to comply with the Security Rule. It also permits a covered entity to change its policies and procedures as long as the changes are documented and implemented in compliance with the Security Rule. The Security Rule does not define a policy or procedure, although policies often set forth an organization's approach and reflect its mission and culture (such as workforce expectations, decision-making responsibilities, and consequences for work rule violations). Procedures generally describe how an organization will carry out its approach via explicit step-by-step instructions. The Security Rule's flexibility allows organizations to follow its own business practices as it develops its policies and procedures (HHS 2007d).

Documentation (45 CFR 164.316(b)(1))

The documentation standard (three implementation specifications, all required) states that covered entities are to "(i) maintain … policies and procedures … in written (which

FIGURE 4.6.	Policies and procedures and documentation requirements		
Standards	**Sections**	**Implementation Specifications** **(R) = Required, (A) = Addressable**	
Policies and Procedures	§ 164.316(a)		
Documentation	§ 164.316(b)(1)	Time Limit	**(R)**
		Availability	**(R)**
		Updates	**(R)**

Source: HHS 2007d

may be electronic) form; and (ii) if an action, activity, or assessment is required … to be documented, maintain a written (which may be electronic) record of the action, activity, or assessment" (45 CFR 164.316(b)(1)). There are three implementation specifications. All are required.

Time Limit (45 CFR 164.316(b)(2)(i))

The first implementation specification, time limit (required), states that covered entities are to "retain the documentation required … for 6 years from the date of its creation or the date when it last was in effect, whichever is later" (45 CFR 164.316(b)(2)(i)). This is a minimum retention period. Organizations may choose or be required to retain documentation longer depending on state statutes or regulations, accreditation standards, or for operational purposes (HHS 2007d). The following example demonstrates how this requirement would be applied: a hospital's policy and procedure went into effect January 1, 2010. It remained in effect until March 1, 2011 when it was substantially changed. The original version would have to be retained in either paper or electronic form until March 1, 2017 (which is six years from the date it was last in effect). The hospital has the freedom to decide how and where the policy and procedure will be retained, but it must be able to produce it if it needs to (Rinehart-Thompson 2011).

Availability (45 CFR 164.316(b)(2)(ii))

The second implementation specification, availability (required), states that documentation must be "available to those persons responsible for implementing the procedures to which the documentation pertains" (45 CFR 164.316(b)(1)(ii)). Ways to carry this out are through printed manuals or websites (HHS 2007d). Policy and procedure documentation related to Security Rule compliance (for example, disciplinary procedures for Security Rule violations and workforce training requirements) cannot be maintained in an administrative office that is inaccessible to those who must carry out the policies and procedures. As documentation becomes increasingly centralized through electronic mechanisms, this requirement should become less of a burden to many organizations.

Updates (45 CFR 164.316(b)(2)(iii))

The third and final implementation specification, updates (required), states that covered entities must "review documentation periodically, and update as needed, in response to environmental or operational changes affecting the security of ePHI" (45 CFR 164.316(b)(1)(iii)). When deciding how frequently to review its documentation, an organization must be aware of the rate at which changes affecting ePHI are occurring. Despite the frequency deemed necessary, documentation must reflect the current status of an organization's HIPAA-compliant security plans and procedures. For example, a hospital's health information department may transition its release-of-information function from a paper-based system to an electronic system. PHI (and information about the release of PHI) that was formerly in paper form is now ePHI. Policies and procedures must be updated to reflect the change in media and to ensure that the ePHI is now safeguarded per HIPAA Security Rule requirements.

CHECK YOUR UNDERSTANDING 4.3

Instructions: Indicate whether the following statements are true or false (T or F).

1. The administrative safeguard standard's termination procedure can be applied to workforce members whose access levels change due to a job description change.

2. The security awareness and training standard emphasizes that a security safeguard cannot completely protect ePHI without the workforce being aware of its responsibilities.

3. The data backup plan and disaster recovery plan implementation specifications are both part of the Security Rule's contingency plan standard.

4. One of the Security Rule's organizational requirement standards states that covered entities must have contracts or other types of arrangements with business associates with access to the covered entity's ePHI.

5. All documentation related to the Security Rule may be retained a maximum of six years.

REAL-WORLD CASE

Chapter 4 discusses many mechanisms to safeguard ePHI. Although many are the responsibility of administration and information technology staff, others fall squarely on the shoulders of each member of the workforce. An example of the latter is the creation of passwords. By creating and updating passwords in a manner that promotes security (and which are often compelled by system requirements), ePHI can be protected at the grassroots level by each and every employee. Because passwords are ubiquitous, their significance in either protecting or exposing ePHI is often overlooked. The following scenario demonstrates how a password can evolve from a low-security, easily decoded one to a password that is deemed robust (and yet easy to recall).

Noel works with ePHI. He is instructed to create a new password to access the information system. He would like to make the process easy for himself, so he decides to use the name of his beloved cat, Dexter. The system rejects this as not being robust enough because the use of a pet's name is a fairly popular option and readily deciphered. Using cues provided by the system, Noel creates a robust password that he may still easily remember, but which is much less easily decoded. Interspersing letters (both upper-case and lower-case), symbols, and numbers, and recognizing that the system requires a minimum of 8 characters, his resulting password is Dex05Ter98! The 05 and 98 represent the month and year that Noel's cat was born. This is easy for Noel to remember because it is meaningful to him, but difficult for others to decipher or decode, even if they know that Noel's cat is named Dexter (Rinehart-Thompson 2011).

A robust system will also require passwords to be periodically changed. However, with periodic changes (particularly if they are scheduled frequently) comes the additional risk that passwords will be posted on computer monitors via post-it notes or written on pieces of paper that can become lost or stolen. Noel wants to be sure this does not happen. When he changes his password, he creates a logical system for himself that is not readily known by others. He uses the name of his beloved deceased cat, Comet. Using the same mechanism that the system accepted when he created his first password, his resulting password is Co07Met98! The system may not allow him to use the final three characters of 98! again. If it does not, he will need to revise the password in a way that is still meaningful to him.

When Noel is required to change his password a third time, he may revert to using the name and birthdate of a childhood pet, applying the same logic that he used to create his first two passwords while using information and a pattern that very few (if any) other people would know. As a result, both Noel and the system are satisfied and the ePHI accessible on his computer is secure.

SUMMARY

The HIPAA Security Rule governs the protection of electronic protected health information. It consisted of five sets of safeguard standards and requirements: physical safeguards (45 CFR 164.310); technical safeguards (45 CFR 164.312); administrative safeguards (45 CFR 164.308); organizational requirements (45 CFR 164.314); and policies and procedures and documentation (45 CFR 164.316). From this chapter, the reader should understand required vs. addressable standards and implementation specifications. The reader should also understand the specific mechanisms that the Security Rule sets forth to safeguard electronic PHI both during transmission and at rest.

REFERENCES

American Health Information Management Association. 2012. *Pocket Glossary for Health Information Management and Technology*, 3rd ed. Chicago: AHIMA.

Brodnik, M, L. Rinehart-Thompson, and R. Reynolds. 2012. *Fundamentals of Law for Health Informatics and Information Management*. Chicago: AHIMA.

Cazier, J. and D. Medlin. 2006. How Secure Is Your Information System? An Investigation into Actual Healthcare Worker Password Practices. *Perspectives in Health Information Management* (3)7.

Department of Health and Human Services. 2012. Health Information Privacy. Breaches Affecting 500 or More Individuals. http://www.hhs.gov/ocr/privacy/hipaa/administrative/breachnotificationrule/breachtool.html.

Department of Health and Human Services. 2007a. HIPAA Security Series: 2-Security Standards: Administrative Safeguards 2(2). http://www.hhs.gov/ocr/privacy/hipaa/administrative/securityrule/adminsafeguards.pdf.

Department of Health and Human Services. 2007b. HIPAA Security Series: 3-Security Standards: Physical Safeguards 2(3). http://www.hhs.gov/ocr/privacy/hipaa/administrative/securityrule/physsafeguards.pdf.

Department of Health and Human Services. 2007c. HIPAA Security Series: 4-Security Standards: Technical Safeguards 2(4). http://www.hhs.gov/ocr/privacy/hipaa/administrative/securityrule/techsafeguards.pdf.

Department of Health and Human Services. 2007d. HIPAA Security Series: 5-Organizational, policies and procedures and documentation requirements 2(5). http://www.hhs.gov/ocr/privacy/hipaa/administrative/securityrule/pprequirements.pdf.

Rinehart-Thompson, L. 2011. AHIMA E-Learning Exam Prep Course: CHPS Domain 3—Information Technology/Physical and Technical Safeguards.

Wager, Karen, Francis Lee, and John Glaser. 2009. *Managing Healthcare Information Systems: A Practical Approach for Healthcare Executives.* San Francisco: Jossey-Bass.

45 CFR 164.302-.318: Security Standards for the Protection of Electronic Protected Health Information. 2006.

45 CFR 164.304: Definitions. 2006.

45 CFR 164.306(a): General Requirements. 2006.

45 CFR 164.306(b): Flexibility of Approach. 2006.

45 CFR 164.306(d): Implementation Specifications. 2006.

45 CFR 164.308: Administrative Safeguards. 2006.

45 CFR 164.308(a)(1)(i): Security Management Process. 2006.

45 CFR 164.308(a)(1)(ii)(A): Risk Analysis. 2006.

45 CFR 164.308(a)(1)(ii)(B): Risk Management. 2006.

45 CFR 164.308(a)(1)(ii)(C): Sanction Policy. 2006.

45 CFR 164.308(a)(1)(ii)(D): Information System Activity Review. 2006.

45 CFR 164.308(a)(2): Assigned Security Responsibility. 2006.

45 CFR 164.308(a)(3)(i): Workforce Security. 2006.

45 CFR 164.308(a)(3)(ii)(A): Authorization and/or Supervision. 2006.

45 CFR 164.308(a)(3)(ii)(B): Workforce Clearance Procedures. 2006.

45 CFR 164.308(a)(3)(ii)(C): Termination Procedures. 2006.

45 CFR 164.308(a)(4)(i): Information Access Management. 2006.

45 CFR 164.308(a)(4)(ii)(A): Isolating Healthcare Clearinghouse Functions. 2006.

45 CFR 164.308(a)(4)(ii)(B): Access Authorization. 2006.

45 CFR 164.308(a)(4)(ii)(C): Access Establishment and Modification. 2006.

45 CFR 164.308(a)(5)(i): Security Awareness and Training. 2006.

45 CFR 164.308(a)(5)(ii)(A): Security Reminders. 2006.

45 CFR 164.308(a)(5)(ii)(B): Protection from Malicious Software. 2006.

45 CFR 164.308(a)(5)(ii)(C): Log-In Monitoring. 2006.

45 CFR 164.308(a)(5)(ii)(D): Password Management. 2006.

45 CFR 164.308(a)(6)(i): Security Incident Procedures. 2006.

45 CFR 164.308(a)(6)(ii): Response and Reporting. 2006.

45 CFR 164.308(a)(7)(i): Contingency Plan. 2006.

45 CFR 164.308(a)(7)(ii)(A): Data Backup Plan. 2006.

45 CFR 164.308(a)(7)(ii)(B): Disaster Recovery Plan. 2006.

45 CFR 164.308(a)(7)(ii)(C): Emergency Mode Operation Plan. 2006.

45 CFR 164.308(a)(7)(ii)(D): Testing and Revision Procedures. 2006.

45 CFR 164.308(a)(7)(ii)(E): Applications and Data Criticality Analysis. 2006.

45 CFR 164.308(a)(8): Evaluation. 2006.

45 CFR 164.308(b)(1): Business Associate Contracts and Other Arrangements. 2006.

45 CFR 164.308(b)(4): Written Contract or Other Arrangement. 2006.

45 CFR 164.310: Physical Safeguards. 2006.

45 CFR 164.310(a)(1): Facility Access Controls. 2006.

45 CFR 164.310(a)(2)(i): Contingency Operations. 2006.

45 CFR 164.310(a)(2)(ii): Facility Security Plan. 2006.

45 CFR 164.310(a)(2)(iii): Access Control and Validation Procedures. 2006.

45 CFR 164.310(a)(2)(iv): Maintenance Records. 2006.

45 CFR 164.310(b): Workstation Use. 2006.

45 CFR 164.310(c): Workstation Security. 2006.

45 CFR 164.310(d)(1): Device and Media Controls. 2006.

45 CFR 164.310(d)(2)(i): Disposal. 2006.

45 CFR 164.310(d)(2)(ii): Media Re-Use. 2006.

45 CFR 164.310(d)(2)(iii): Accountability. 2006.

45 CFR 164.310(d)(2)(iv): Data Backup and Storage. 2006.

45 CFR 164.312: Technical Safeguards. 2006.

45 CFR 164.312(a)(1): Access Control. 2006.

45 CFR 164.312(a)(2)(i): Unique User Identification. 2006.

45 CFR 164.312(a)(2)(ii): Emergency Access Procedure. 2006.

45 CFR 164.312(a)(2)(iii): Automatic Log-Off. 2006.

45 CFR 164.312(a)(2)(iv): Encryption and Decryption. 2006.

45 CFR 164.312(b): Audit Controls. 2006.

45 CFR 164.312(c)(1): Integrity. 2006.

45 CFR 164.312(c)(2): Mechanism to Authenticate Electronic Protected Health Information. 2006.

45 CFR 164.312(d): Person or Entity Authentication. 2006.

45 CFR 164.312(e)(1): Transmission Security. 2006.

45 CFR 164.312(e)(2)(i): Integrity Controls. 2006.

45 CFR 164.312(e)(2)(ii): Encryption. 2006.

45 CFR 164.314: Organizational Requirements. 2006.

45 CFR 164.314(a)(1): Business Associate Contracts or Other Arrangements. 2006

45 CFR 164.314(a)(2)(i): Business Associate Contracts. 2006.

45 CFR 164.314(a)(2)(ii): Other Arrangements. 2006.

45 CFR 164.314(b)(1): Requirements for Group Health Plans. 2006.

45 CFR 164.314(b)(2): Implementation Specifications. 2006.

45 CFR 164.316: Policies and Procedures and Documentation Requirements. 2006.

45 CFR 164.316(a): Policies and Procedures. 2006.

45 CFR 164.316(b)(1): Documentation. 2006.

45 CFR 164.316(b)(2)(i): Time Limit. 2006.

45 CFR 164.316(b)(2)(ii): Availability. 2006.

45 CFR 164.316(b)(2)(iii): Updates. 2006.

164.504(f)(2)(iii): Requirements for Plan Documents. 2006.

CHAPTER 5

Threat Identification, Risk Analysis, and Disaster Recovery/Business Continuity

Learning Objectives

- Explain the concepts of risk analysis and risk management

- Give examples of human threats and natural and environmental threats

- Explain the purpose and descibe the steps of a risk analysis

- Distinguish a disaster recovery plan from a contingency plan

- Explain the purpose of a disaster recovery plan and a contingency plan

- Identify the HIPAA Security Rule requirements for a disaster recovery plan and contingency plan

- Describe mechanisms for backup and recovering data

- Describe the steps for implementing an emergency mode of operations for unplanned situations

- Describe the steps for developing a business continuity plan

- Discuss security concerns associated with health information exchanges and other arrangements where electronic PHI is transmitted

KEY TERMS

Business continuity plan

Contingency plan

Control analysis

Control recommendations

Core operations

Creditor

Data backup

Data recovery

Disaster recovery plan

E-mail

Emergency mode of operations

External threats

Facsimile (fax)

Fair and Accurate Credit Transaction Act (FACTA)

General support systems

Health Information Exchange (HIE)

Impact analysis

Internal threats

Likelihood determination

Major applications

Medical identity theft

Patient Portal

Personal Health Record (PHR)

Personal Health Record Portal

Record locator service (RLS)

Red flags

Red Flags Rule

Regional Health Information Organization (RHIO)

Residual risks

Risk determination

System characterization

Telemedicine

Text messaging

Vulnerability

INTRODUCTION

Conducting business involves risks, which can threaten an organization in many different ways. Although it is not possible to completely eliminate risks, a business can and should take steps to identify its risks and take steps to control them so the resulting damage—both financially and to an organization's reputation—is minimized. Chapter 4 described how the HIPAA Security Rule requires covered entities to conduct a risk analysis to safeguard its electronic protected health information (ePHI).

This chapter discusses risk identification by outlining the steps involved in conducting a risk analysis. It further discusses what an organization can do to prepare for the possibility of a risk becoming a reality through the development of disaster recovery and business continuity plans that safeguard the availability, confidentiality, and integrity of health information. These steps apply to all business operations, but this chapter will view them primarily through the lens of protecting individuals' health information.

Section 1: Risk Analysis and Management Overview

There are two primary steps in addressing the risks that businesses, including healthcare organizations, face. The first is to analyze them through a risk analysis. The second is to decide, if a risk becomes a reality, how to proceed with operations through disaster recovery and business continuity planning. The next section describes the first step, risk analysis.

The HIPAA Security Rule, which applies to ePHI, requires a risk analysis. The requirement applies not only to covered entities and business associates, but also to agents and subcontractors of business associates (Walsh 2011). The administrative safeguards state that a risk analysis consists of "an accurate and thorough assessment of the potential risks and vulnerabilities to the confidentiality, integrity, and availability" of ePHI (45 CFR 164.308(a)(1)(ii)(A)). After the risks associated with the protection of ePHI have been assessed, an organization must implement a risk management process to "reduce risks and vulnerabilities to a reasonable and appropriate level" (45 CFR 164.308(a)(1)(ii)(B)). The Security Rule frequently uses the terms "reasonable" and "appropriate," but they are not defined. This is due, in part, to the fact that what is reasonable and appropriate will differ from one organization to the next.

Section 2: Risk Analysis Framework

The HIPAA Security Rule does not mandate how a risk analysis should be carried out. However, recognized risk analysis steps are outlined in this sections. Note: although the Security Rule applies only to ePHI, processes should be in place to safeguard all types of PHI, including paper.

System Characterization

The first step of risk analysis is **system characterization**. It focuses on what the organization possesses by identifying which information assets need protection. The assets may be identified either because they are critical to business operations (for example, the data itself, such as ePHI) or because critical data is processed and stored on the system (such as hardware). The greatest focus should be placed on the assets identified as the most critical. This determination can be made by identifying which assets have the greatest effect on the organization's operations and which assets create the greatest risk to the organization if they are not functional. Using these factors, assets can be ranked by relative criticality (Walsh 2011).

To make sure that no assets are missed, identification should include a complete inventory of **major applications** (that is, those that are critical to the organization or that store PHI) and **general support systems** (namely, any system that stores or processes ePHI). Generally, a major application is "owned" by the director of a department that primarily uses that application. For example, a laboratory director would be the "owner" of the laboratory information system. The owner of the electronic health record (EHR) is more likely to vary from one organization to another. In one organization, it may be the chief operating officer. In another organization, it may be the director of health information services. The IT department generally owns general support systems, which includes computer workstations, laptops and tablets, mobile devices, networks, and e-mail systems (Walsh 2011).

Once system characterization has been completed, an organization has to identify three elements to decide how likely it is that an event will occur given the organization's current status. These elements are the threats themselves (also known as threat sources), vulnerabilities, and controls that the organization has in place to inhibit the threats (NIST 2002). These three elements are outlined in the next three subsections.

Identifying Threats

After major applications and general support systems have been identified and ranked, the second step in risk analysis is to look at what might threaten an organization's assets. Threats can impact many types of organizational information (for example, supply inventory and payroll). The focus of this text is health information, however, where threats to its security can compromise confidentiality, integrity, and availability. It is important to identify those potential threats (Walsh 2011). An organization should focus on threats that might be reasonably anticipated rather than accounting for every possible threat. Reasonably anticipated threats may be identified based on factors such as an organization's past experiences, its geographic characteristics, and industry trends. Once threats are identified, they should be mapped to the major applications and general support systems. For example, one type of threat (theft) should be mapped to mobile devices.

Health information can be threatened by humans as well as by natural and environmental factors. Threats posed by humans can be either unintentional or intentional. Threats to health information can result in compromised integrity (that is, alteration of information, either intentional or unintentional), theft (intentional by nature), loss (unintentional) or intentional misplacement, other wrongful uses or disclosures (either intentional or unintentional), and destruction (intentional or unintentional) (Rinehart-Thompson 2011). Many of these incidents constitute a breach, as defined by HITECH. Human threats and natural and environmental threats can be either internal or external. This text will describe threats as internal or external, thereafter discussing human as well as natural and environmental threats that can occur within each category. **Internal threats** to information privacy and security are those that originate within an organization. **External threats** to information privacy and security are those that originate outside an organization.

Internal Threats

Humans are the most constant threat to health information integrity. Whether intentional or unintentional, incidents resulting from internal human threats are more common than incidents resulting from external human threats because individuals within an organization often have constant access to large amounts of information. Because intentional breaches are often committed by disgruntled employees, organizations should avoid offering employment with access to patient information to individuals who often change jobs. Temporary or short-term contract employees pose a greater internal threat because their limited commitment to the organization may make them less loyal more difficult to locate after an incident has occurred. Also, if they do not hold a license or professional credential, they will not face sanctions affecting their professional status. Threats to paper records include unauthorized access and photocopying.

Although internal threats often affect the security of information in an organization's system, they also include the installation and use of unauthorized software, introduction of computer viruses, and use of an organization's computer equipment for unauthorized or illegal activities. These include accessing pornographic sites or other sites the organization does not authorize, harassing or soliciting others via e-mail, or carrying on a business for personal profit by using an organization's computer equipment (Rinehart-Thompson 2011).

Internal natural and environmental factors can also threaten health information by compromising or destroying it. Electrical disruptions, fire, flooding, or other water damage that originates within the organization are all examples of internal natural and environmental threats (Rinehart-Thompson 2011).

External Threats

External human threats are not as prevalent as internal human threats, but they tend to be intentional because of the effort they require. Computer hackers or other computer-savvy individuals may threaten a system and its data. Examples of intentional external threats caused by humans include intentional alteration of information, theft of information, intentional misplacement of information, and intentional destruction of information. Humans can introduce computer viruses into a system from external sources such as emails or attachments to program files loaded onto a system (Rinehart-Thompson 2011).

External natural and environmental threats can also threaten health information by compromising or destroying it. Power surges or failures, fire, tornadoes, lightning, earthquakes, storms, hurricanes, and flooding or other types of water damage that originate outside the organization are all examples of external natural and environmental threats.

Medical Identity Theft

One type of intentional threat to health information is **medical identity theft**. A subset of identity theft, it involves the "inappropriate or unauthorized misrepresentation of one's identity, generally without the individual's knowledge or permission, to (1) obtain medical services or goods, or (2) obtain money by falsifying claims for medical services and falsifying medical records to support those claims" (Dixon 2006). In some cases, however, the person whose identity has been misrepresented may actually have given consent, but perhaps without a full understanding of the consequences. For example, an insured individual may allow an uninsured friend or family member to use the insured's medical insurance card so medical services will be covered. If a patient's financial information is used to purchase nonmedical goods or services, this is not medical identity theft because the consequences are financial only. For example, if a hospital business office employee uses her position to access a patient's information, including the patient's credit card number, and assumes the patient's identity to go on a shopping spree to purchase jewelry, this is not medical identity theft (Rinehart-Thompson 2011).

Medical identity theft differs from financial identity theft because both the victim's financial status *and* medical information are negatively impacted. While financial identity theft victims may face financial consequences (such as monetary loss, damaged credit, or debt collection efforts), medical identity theft victims face financial and other consequences, including insurance denials (if lifetime caps are reached), and improper and potentially life-threatening medical treatment once medical information about the perpetrator is intertwined with the victim's in the victim's health record (Rinehart-Thompson 2011).

As with threats to health information generally, medical identity theft can also be categorized as internal or external. Internal medical identity theft is committed by an organization's insiders, namely staff who can access patient information. Individuals may be employees who act alone or imposters who obtain employment and pose as staff while their main purpose is to steal patient-identifying information as members of sophisticated crime rings. They continue in their roles until they are caught or complete what they intended to, leaving the organization while their activities have yet to be noticed. Where PHI is electronic, large amounts of patient information can be accessed and downloaded at one time.

Ways to deter internal medical identity theft include adequate pre-employment screens and ongoing background checks (Rinehart-Thompson 2011).

External medical identity theft is committed by individuals outside an organization. It includes uninsured individuals who assume another's identity based on need (as described previously). Baseline identification (for example, taking pictures of patients at the time of registration or scanning drivers' licenses) is often used to deter external medical identity theft. Organizations must develop separate mechanisms to combat internal and external medical identity theft because the perpetrators in each type differ greatly. Individuals internal to an organization must be screened and monitored to prevent and detect internal medical identity theft. Conversely, individuals seeking treatment must be screened to prevent and detect external medical identity theft.

Breaches

The HITECH definition of breach is the "unauthorized acquisition, access, use, or disclosure of PHI which compromises the security or privacy of such information" (ARRA 2009). Although this concept will be discussed in detail in chapter 6, it is important to note here that medical identity theft incidents will often fit the breach definition. If a covered entity, business associate, or subcontractor commits a breach, it must follow HIPAA breach notification requirements.

Red Flags Rule

In December 2010, the **Fair and Accurate Credit Transaction Act (FACTA)**, a federal statute that protects consumers with regard to their credit (for example, by allowing annual free credit reports), was amended to address identity theft issues. The amendment, the **Red Flags Rule**, requires financial institutions and creditors to develop and implement written identity theft programs in an effort to identify, detect, and respond to **red flags**, which are indicators that trigger the presence of potential identity theft. The law does not address medical identity theft, but many healthcare organizations are creditors. As defined by the law, a **creditor** is anyone:

> …who regularly, and in the ordinary course of business: obtains or uses consumer reports in connection with a credit transaction; furnishes information to consumer reporting agencies in connection with a credit transaction; or advances funds to—or on behalf of— someone, except for funds for expenses incidental to a service provided by the creditor to that person. (FTC n.d.)

This definition was updated after the American Medical Association (AMA), speaking on behalf of physicians and other organizations, disputed a previous broader definition of creditor. The AMA successfully argued that it was improper to treat physician practices similarly to banks and other financial institutions (Rinehart-Thompson 2011).

The Federal Trade Commission issued and enforces the Red Flags Rule. The enforcement date was December 31, 2010. The five red flags categories are:

- Alerts, notifications, or other warnings received from consumer reporting agencies or service providers, such as fraud detection services

- The presentation of suspicious documents

- The presentation of suspicious personally identifying information, such as a suspicious address change

- The unusual use of, or other suspicious activity related to, a covered account

- Notices from customers, victims of identity theft, law enforcement authorities, or other persons regarding possible identity theft in connection with covered accounts held by the financial institution or creditor (FTC 2007)

Even if a healthcare provider does not meet the Red Flags Rule definition of a creditor, the World Privacy Forum recommends that it incorporates red flags related to patients and insurers into their policies and procedures for preventing, detecting, and mitigating identity theft (Gellman and Dixon 2009).

Identifying Vulnerabilities

After an organization has characterized its system (step 1) and threats have been identified (step 2), the third step in a risk analysis plan is to identify vulnerabilities.

A **vulnerability** is "an inherent weakness or absence of a safeguard that could be exploited by a threat" (Walsh 2011). An example of an inherent weakness is the absence of antivirus software on an organization's information system or the presence of antivirus software that is not regularly updated (Walsh 2011). One threat source may exploit more than one vulnerability. For example, a disgruntled terminated employee (a threat source) whose access has not been disabled may exploit both an absence of antivirus software and a less-than-robust firewall (both vulnerabilities). One vulnerability may be exploited by multiple threats. For example, a computer hacker and a disgruntled terminated employee who still has access to a system represent two different types of threats. An absence of antivirus software (a vulnerability) could be exploited by both of these threats. On the other hand, one control (such as installing antivirus software) may be implemented to stop multiple threats from occurring (Walsh 2011). If a vulnerability is exploited, potential losses include tangible assets and an organization's reputation (Rinehart-Thompson 2011). It is important for an organization to identify its vulnerabilities so they can be controlled.

Control Analysis

The fourth step in risk analysis is **control analysis**. It goes hand-in-hand with vulnerability identification as it looks at ways that an organization controls its vulnerabilities to threats with the goal of eliminating or at least reducing the likelihood that a threat will successfully take advantage of a vulnerability (NIST 2002). There are five categories of controls and they are outlined in figure 5.1. Controls in the five categories can generally be identified as technical (for example, mechanisms that are part of the system software or hardware (such as firewalls) or nontechnical (for example, policies and procedures designed to guide employee behavior) (NIST 2002).

FIGURE 5.1.	Categories of controls	
Type	**Action**	**Examples**
Preventive	Inhibits a threat	Access controls, encryption
Deterrent	Keeps casual threats away	Strong passwords
Detective	Identifies and proves when a threat has occurred or might occur	Audit trails, intrusion detection
Reactive	Responds to a threat that has occurred	Alarms
Recovery	Helps retrieve or recreate data or applications	Backup systems, contingency plans

Source: Walsh 2011

In addition to control analysis, there are other ways to identify vulnerabilities. These can take place in the form of "lessons learned" from other organizations, such as reviewing the Department of Health and Human Services' website of breaches affecting 500 or more individuals (HHS 2012), searching the Internet, or scanning the news for data breaches. They can also take place internally through activities such as looking at past incidents or data breaches; conducting internal audits, or arranging for audits by external auditors; conducting walk-through inspections; reviewing patient complaints regarding security shortcomings; conducting privacy and security gap analyses; and performing network vulnerability scans (Walsh 2011).

Likelihood Determination

In determining the amount of resources to dedicate toward potential threats, an organization needs to consider two major factors: (1) how likely is it that a particular threat will actually occur and, (2) if it does occur, how great will its impact or severity be? The fifth step in a risk analysis, **likelihood determination**, considers the first factor. As stated in step 2, identifying threats, an organization needs to focus on events that it might reasonably expect. Once identified, they are categorized based on the likelihood or probability that they will exploit the organization's vulnerabilities. For example, an organization might determine that inappropriate access to health information by its employees is more likely than a system disruption resulting from a tornado. An organization's security safeguards and controls must be considered in conjunction with the likelihood (Walsh 2011). Figure 5.2 demonstrates the definition of each likelihood level.

FIGURE 5.2.	Likelihood levels and definitions
Likelihood Level	**Likelihood Definition**
High	Threat source is highly motivated and sufficiently capable, and controls to prevent vulnerability are ineffective
Medium	Threat source is motivated and capable, but controls that are in place may impede successful exercise of vulnerability
Low	Threat source lacks motivation or capability, or controls are in place to prevent or significantly impede the vulnerability from being exploited

Source: Walsh 2011

Impact Analysis

The sixth step in a risk analysis is **impact analysis**, which is considering how great a threat's impact might be. An organization must anticipate, if a threat source successfully exploits an organization's vulnerabilities, how significantly it will affect the organization (NIST 2002). For example, an organization might determine that a system disruption resulting from a tornado would have a greater impact than inappropriate access to health information by employees. Figure 5.3 illustrates the impact levels and their definitions.

FIGURE 5.3.	Impact levels and definitions
Magnitude of Impact	**Impact Definition**
High	Exploitation of vulnerability • May result in high costly loss of major tangible assets or resources; • May violate, harm, or impede an organization's mission, reputation, or interest significantly; or • May result in human death or serious injury

(Continued on next page)

FIGURE 5.3.	(Continued)
Magnitude of Impact	**Impact Definition**
Medium	Exploitation of vulnerability • May result in costly loss of tangible assets or resources; • May violate, harm, or impede an organization's mission, reputation, or interest; or • May result in human injury
Low	Exploitation of vulnerability • May result in loss of some tangible assets or resources; or • May affect an organization's mission, reputation, or interest noticeably

Source: Walsh 2011

Risk Determination

The seventh step is **risk determination**. This occurs after steps 5 and 6 have been completed. This step considers how likely is it that a particular threat will actually occur and, if it does occur, how great its impact or severity will be. Risk determination quantifies an organization's threats and enables it to both prioritize its risks and appropriately allocate its limited resources (namely, people, time, and money) accordingly. In the risk determination process, scores are assigned to risks based on the risk's likelihood (determined in step 5) and impact (determined in step 6). In the first method, a qualitative approach, the likelihood and impact scores are multiplied. The second method, a quantitative approach, implements a cost-benefit analysis of potential controls that an organization might use (NIST 2002). Both approaches are described in figure 5.4. Examples of each are provided in figure 5.5.

Control Recommendations

The eighth step, **control recommendations**, assesses how an organization can deal with a vulnerability when it does not have a control in place. For example, a vulnerability would be the lack of a procedure to disable employee access to an information system before they are notified of their termination. A control recommendation would be to implement such a procedure. Not all vulnerabilities have control recommendations (Rinehart-Thompson 2011).

Results Documentation

Step nine is results documentation. It is important to document risk analysis reports, which include findings of key vulnerabilities and control recommendations (as described in step eight). Standard formats include spreadsheets and summary reports. Risk profiles should be created for areas that present risks (for example, computer workstations). The organization should also be aware of **residual risks**, which are risks that continue to exist even after the organization has applied safeguards and controls (Walsh 2011). HIPAA does not specify the format of documentation, but it does require that risk analysis documentation be retained for six years.

FIGURE 5.4.	Qualitative and quantitative approaches to risk determination
Qualitative Approach	Likelihood and effect are rated as high (3), medium (2), or low (1). The values assigned to each (likelihood and effect) are multiplied for a combined score.
Quantitative Approach	Monetary values are assigned to potential losses. Factors to be considered include: • Value of asset being protected • Estimate of frequency of threat across time • Approximate cost (measurable and intangible) of each occurrence

Source: Walsh 2011

FIGURE 5.5.	Examples of qualitative and quantitative approaches to risk determination		
Quantitative Approach (Risk = Likelihood × Effect)			
		Effect	
		Low	**Medium**	**High**
Likelihood	High	3	6	9
	Medium	2	4	6
	Low	1	2	3

Quantitative Approach

If an organization estimates an annual loss of $5,000, a control that costs $20,000 will pay for itself in 4 years. If an update or replacement of the control is needed within that time period, however, it may be more cost-effective to simply address the cost of the risk that is causing the loss rather than implementing the control. However, this would depend on the cost of updating and replacing the control.

Source: Walsh 2011

CHECK YOUR UNDERSTANDING 5.1

Instructions: Indicate whether the following statements are true or false (T or F).

1. General support systems store or process ePHI.
2. Human threats to the integrity of health information are always internal.
3. Individuals who commit internal medical identity theft may be part of a crime ring.
4. The definition of "creditor" under the Red Flags Rule was written to include as many physicians as possible.
5. In an impact analysis, a threat with a medium impact magnitude may result in human death or serious injury.

Section 3: Contingency and Disaster Recovery Plans

This chapter has discussed the steps an organization should take to prepare for the possibility of a threat becoming an actual event. Although smaller events such as short-term power outages will cause only minimal disruptions, organizations must plan for large-scale events (disasters) such as tornadoes and floods that have the potential to significantly disrupt operations for indefinite periods of time. An organization must prepare for both, determining how it will recover from an event and continue to operate. This section discusses the steps an organization should take once an event does occur, both in the short term and in the long term.

An organization's plans must address every aspect of an organization's operations (for example, a hospital must address the continuation of medical services as part of its plan). Inherent in these plans are the protection of health information and the continuation of operations that affect health information. If planned appropriately, a contingency plan and its disaster recovery plan will "secure health information from damage, ensure stability in continuity of care activities, and provide for orderly recovery of information" (AHIMA 2010a).

Contingency Plan

A **contingency plan** is a documented set of procedures for responding to emergencies. It includes operating during and after an event that limits or prevents access to facilities and patient information so at least a limited level of service can be provided. This may include arranging for the use of alternative facilities (AHIMA 2012a). Thereafter, it includes the continuation of services through a business continuity plan, which is discussed later in this chapter. The ultimate goal of a contingency plan is to return to normal operations as quickly as possible. Contingency plan is an umbrella term that addresses what an organization and its personnel will do both during and after event. Thus, it also encompasses the disaster recovery plan and business continuity and emergency mode of operations, described in the following sections. All three types of plans, of course, must be prepared before an event occurs.

Once an event is over and operations have returned to normal, meetings with staff are necessary to evaluate what worked well and what did not in the overall contingency plan and its execution. These lessons learned allow for procedural updates so that future events will create less disruption.

The term *contingency* appears in two separate sections of the HIPAA Security Rule: in the seventh administrative safeguard (of nine) and in the first physical safeguard (of four). Figure 5.6 demonstrates this, in addition to the term *emergency mode operation*, which is discussed later in this chapter. Naturally, these provisions address the safeguarding and restoration of ePHI.

FIGURE 5.6.	HIPAA Security Rule requirements for contingency and disaster recovery planning	
Safeguard Standard		**Implementation Specification**
Administrative	Contingency plan (45 CFR 164.308(a)(7))	Disaster recovery plan (required): must include procedures to restore any lost data
		Emergency mode operation plan (required): must have procedures that provide for the continuation of critical business processes needed to protect ePHI while operating in emergency mode
Physical	Facility access controls (45 CFR164.310(a)(1))	Contingency operations (addressable): should have procedures to allow facility access to support the restoration of lost data under the disaster recovery plan and emergency mode operations plan

Disaster Recovery Plan

An immediate component of a contingency plan is the **disaster recovery plan**, which defines the resources, actions, tasks, and data required to restore critical services as quickly as possible and manage business recovery processes after an event has occurred (AHIMA 2012a). The term *disaster recovery plan* appears as an implementation specification in the administrative safeguard contingency plan standard of the HIPAA Security Rule. Figure 5.6 demonstrates this. This provision, too, addresses the safeguarding and restoration of ePHI, which means that preventive actions must be taken to ensure that data is not lost (for example, by routinely making duplicate copies of data), ensuring the confidentiality of the data, and providing for data to be available after an event for users who need it.

Protecting Privacy and Security During Disasters

An important part of contingency and disaster recovery planning is making patient information available while also preserving its confidentiality and integrity.

The privacy and security of patient information must be maintained, whether it exists electronically or on paper. Physical security must be maintained both on-site and at any backup sites. This can be accomplished by securing the premises through mechanisms such as locks and access controls (for examples, key cards or biometric scans) and granting access only to authorized personnel. In addition to these preventative measures, access attempts and successful access can be tracked retrospectively with audit trails. An organization should be able to answer the following questions before an event occurs: how will information be protected during an emergency, and who is responsible for ensuring that data and the systems on which they reside are secure during the emergency (Halpert 2008a)?

After basic functionality has been restored, the most applicable sections of the HIPAA Privacy Rule are managing the facility directory, controlling uses and disclosures of PHI, managing business associate agreements, and creating documentation that will allow patients to continue to exercise their HIPAA individual rights: access to the designated record set, amendment requests, and accounting of disclosures requests (Halpert 2008b).

Business Continuity and Emergency Mode of Operations

Associated with a contingency plan is a **business continuity plan**, which directs an organization via policies and procedures as to how it will continue its business operations during a computer system shutdown (AHIMA 2012a). Similar to a business continuity plan is an **emergency mode of operations**, which describes the processes and controls that will be followed until operations are fully restored following an event (AHIMA 2012a). The intent behind both is to "preserve business in the wake of a disaster or disruption of service" (AHIMA 2012b). The term *emergency mode operation* appears in the administrative safeguard standards of the HIPAA Security Rule. This is displayed in figure 5.6.

Organizations must determine in advance how they will operate in emergency mode (before the interruption is fixed) to continue business operations. They should determine how operations will continue if certain employees cannot work by identifying the minimum number of people (a skeleton staff) needed to complete each function. Alternate plans must be made if there is not enough space for all personnel to work during an emergency. This may include plans for certain staff members to work remotely where possible. Organizations must also determine, if access to information is lost, how it will be obtained.

Staff should be assessed before an emergency situation to ensure they can respond appropriately. Assessment can occur through routine drills. Staff should be able to do things such as locate disaster protocols and emergency phone numbers; verbalize contingency plans and their individual responsibilities for different types of disasters; describe methods that have been developed to protect equipment and information from damage; and describe methods for moving and storing critical equipment and information (AHIMA 2010a).

All business continuity plans and emergency modes of operations should identify **core operations**, which are functions the organization decides must continue despite an event. For example, the health information department may decide that the master patient index and chart tracking functions are core operations because patients must continue to be identified appropriately and information must continue to be available, despite an event. For each core operation, the organization must document what will happen to that operation if certain disruptions occur; which departments will be affected by the disruption; what the alternatives are (likely with limitations) for carrying out that operation; activities that will continue to be completed; and responsible persons. If electronic systems are not functioning, business continuity for health information management includes ensuring documentation on paper occurs, establishing emergency registration that can function as patient identification, using alternative methods to identify allergies and other emergency conditions, and creating manual filing systems (AHIMA 2010a).

Data Management and Recovery

A critical component of business continuity and emergency mode of operations is data. Data management and recovery involve two parts: maintaining the system and the software on which the data resides; and backing up the data so retrieving it is possible and the recovery process is relatively seamless.

System and Software Maintenance

It is important that both a system's hardware and software are maintained to prevent threats from becoming events. Specific threats to a hardware and software were discussed earlier in this chapter in the sections on identifying threats and vulnerabilities. Maintenance also includes data backup and making improvements based on lessons learned following an event.

Data Backup and Recovery

Data backup is a key element of disaster planning. **Data backup** is the copying of data to secondary storage devices. It is associated with electronic information because it is generally not realistic to duplicate paper records solely for data backup purposes (note, though, that some organizations scan records routinely for ease of access, but maintain the original paper records indefinitely). Backed up data is helpful in restoring original data after data loss has occurred. Not only is data backup beneficial; it is also required for organizations bound by HIPAA. The HIPAA Security Rule includes data backup plan (required) as an implementation specification within the contingency plan standard of administrative safeguards. The rule states that an organization must have "procedures to create and maintain retrievable exact copies of ePHI" (45 CFR 164.308(a)(7)(ii)(A)). Once data back-up is complete, electronic data should be reintegrated with paper records.

Data should be backed up routinely to protect against not only catastrophic disruptions such as floods or hurricanes, but also potentially routine events such as power outages.

Data can be backed up on various types of media. These include CD-ROMs, tapes, external hard drives, online backup services, and off-site data backup services. There are also numerous storage options. Movable storage devices can be maintained either on-site or off-site in a secure location. On-site storage is riskier because an event could destroy both the original and the backed up data. Data can also be transferred to remote locations controlled either by the organization itself or by a third party (that is, a business associate). Organizations should research both the longevity and security of third party storage companies, although the latter is to be addressed via a business associate agreement (Rinehart-Thompson 2011).

Data recovery is the retrieval of information that has been lost due to an event. Data recovery efforts should be minimal for electronic information if thorough and consistent data backup and storage methods were followed. Companies exist to recover damaged electronic data. Data recovery for paper records is more complicated. If the damage is not too extensive, smoke-damaged or water-damaged records may be restored via freeze drying. Damaged records may also be scanned to avoid concerns about further deterioration (Rinehart-Thompson 2011).

An entity (contractor) that restores health records, whether electronic or paper, is a business associate. As such, restoration must be compliant with both the HIPAA Privacy and Security Rules. The business associate agreement must include the standard required terms. Statements to be included in the agreement are outlined in figure 5.7.

FIGURE 5.7.	Business associate agreement provisions for data recovery contractors

- Method of recovery
- A statement that the information will not be further used or disclosed except as permitted or required by the contract
- A statement that appropriate safeguards will be used to prevent use or disclosure not permitted by the contract
- A statement that inappropriate uses or disclosures of which the contractor is aware will be reported to the contracting entity
- A statement that subcontractors or agents who access the information will agree to the same restrictions and conditions
- Indemnification for loss resulting from unauthorized disclosure by the contractor
- Return of the information (by the contractor) when the contract ends or, alternatively, a certificate of destruction and assurances by the contractor that no copies were retained
- Time that will elapse between acquisition and return of information and equipment
- Authorization of the contracting entity to terminate the contract due to violation of any material term

Source: AHIMA 2010a

Although recovery of data is the goal, full recovery is not always possible. There are methods for recovering as much data as possible. These include reprinting or uploading data and documents from undamaged databases (for example, transcription and laboratory); retranscribing documents that are still available in dictation systems; obtaining copies of records from entities that received records from the organization (for example, physician offices); and obtaining copies of records from other departments within the organization that were not affected by the event (for example, the business office). The organization should document both successful and unsuccessful recovery and reconstruction efforts. Future disclosures must include documentation about portions of the record that were lost or reconstructed (AHIMA 2010a).

If no data recovery is possible, the date of loss, recovery and reconstruction efforts attempted, information lost, and event that caused the loss should all be documented. A log of lost or destroyed records should be created to assist with future patient requests, as well as inquiries from accreditation organizations and legal entities (AHIMA 2010a).

Section 4: Health Information Security in HIEs, RHIOs, and Other Electronic Transmissions

Health Information Exchanges

Health information exchange (HIE), is a growing concept. AHIMA defines an HIE as "the electronic movement of health-related information among organizations according to nationally recognized standards" (AHIMA 2010b). The movement of health information can occur across organizations, communities, or regions. A number of private and public entities have received federal funds under ARRA to develop statewide HIEs. Although there may be a variety of uses for information transmitted via an HIE, the most commonly anticipated reason is treatment.

Challenges to the privacy and security of information in HIEs result from inconsistent interpretation and application of the HIPAA Privacy and Security Rules; inconsistencies among state privacy laws; inconsistencies between state and federal privacy laws; and a lack of trust (among healthcare organizations competing in the same market, as well as by individuals whose information is included in the HIE).

In some states, security standards are being implemented in the law. For example, state laws may require such measures as audit logs, parameters around who can access data in an HIE, and requirements for user authentication.

There are different models in place for the inclusion of patient information in an HIE. In one model, an individual must have given permission for his information to be included in an HIE. This is the "opt-in" model. Once a decision is made, all information is included or not included, depending on what the individual decided. This is contrasted with the "opt-out" model, which presumes the individual gives his permission to be included in the HIE unless he actively removes himself from it. All information is included or not included. A third model, the "no consent" model, does not allow an individual to opt out. There are also hybrid models, such as variations on the opt-in and opt-out models that allow individuals to decide that some information will be included for exchange in an

HIE, while other information will not. These models require greater sophistication. As a result, many HIEs are not yet able to accommodate this level of specificity. Whichever model is used, it cannot violate state law. The health information of individuals who opt out of an HIE can still be shared among providers for treatment purposes because HIPAA permits this; however, sharing occurs among traditional release-of-information methods such as US mail or faxing (Warner 2011).

The Office of the National Coordinator (ONC), has published "The Nationwide Privacy and Security Framework for Electronic Exchange of Individually Identifiable Health Information." The publication discusses limitations on the type and amount of ePHI that is collected, used, and disclosed, stating that these limitations are key to minimizing the misuse and abuse of information (ONC 2008).

Privacy and security issues associated with HIEs are the responsibility of both the HIE and the organizations participating in the HIE. Management and audit measures must be in place to address these issues. These are addressed in figure 5.8.

FIGURE 5.8.	Privacy and security measures for health information exchanges (HIEs)

HIEs must consider:

- Access control and levels of access
- Breach notification
- Consent and authorization process
- Consumer education to foster trust
- Data loss protection
- Data use and disclosure, including permissible purposes such as treatment, public health uses, healthcare operations uses, and research

Organizations within HIEs must consider:

- How is data ownership defined?
- What information will be exchanged?
- How will access to the information be authorized?
- How will authorization be tracked and controlled?
- How will user access be authenticated?
- How will authentication be tracked and controlled?
- How will access be tracked and controlled?
- What will the retention schedule be for audit logs?
- How will the HIE and its participating organizations communicate with patients (that is, consumers)?
- What terms should be included in a contract between the HIE and participating organizations to ensure protection of patient information shared by the participant?

Source: AHIMA 2011 and LaTour and Eichenwald-Maki 2010

Regional Health Information Organizations

Regional health information organizations (RHIOs) are collaboratives that exchange health information regionally. As opposed to an HIE, which is described as a process, RHIOs are described as groups of organizations that consist of diverse stakeholders such as providers and payers. They are limited to specific regions such as states, regions within states, or communities. They utilize decentralized databases that are linked together by a centralized **record locator service (RLS)** that indicates where a particular patient may have health information, based on probability equations (AHIMA 2012a). Via interfaces, the databases can communicate with each other. Participants can search for patient records on other participants' systems, but the records remain on the system on which they were created. When a patient is located via the RLS, all participating databases are notified that information exists about that patient. This extensive sharing of patient information raises privacy and security issues also experienced by HIEs. The term RHIO has become somewhat obsolete because of the limited geographical boundaries associated with it (Amatayakul 2012).

Personal Health Record Portals

A **patient portal** is an electronic repository of information about a patient that the individual can access by using the Internet. It is often hosted and controlled by a provider or payer. Patients may be able to add health information to a designated area of the portal, but they do not control the portal. Primarily, patients have the ability to view EHR information about themselves.

In contrast, **personal health record portals**, although also accessed through the Internet, allow patients to create and control the content of their own **personal health record (PHR)**. PHRs, although not official business records, can portray a longitudinal account of a patient's health history if the information is diligently recorded. A PHR portal may be hosted by a provider, payer, or other commercial entity (for example, Microsoft, or other lesser known entities).

HITECH states that PHR vendors and third-party service providers of PHR vendors that qualify as business associates are subject to breach notification requirements and penalties. An example of a PHR vendor is a commercial company that sets up and maintains a website where individuals can store their health information in an online repository. An example of a third-party service provider of a PHR vendor is a company that provides PHR applications such as blood sugar test results that individuals can upload into an online PHR. This HITECH provision is discussed in greater detail in chapter 6. PHR vendors and third-party service providers of PHR vendors that are neither covered entities nor business associates are not subject to HITECH's provisions; however, they are required to comply with the Federal Trade Commission's breach notification regulations.

E-mails

Electronic mail or **e-mail** is used for provider-to-provider communication; it is also a way for providers and patients to communicate with each other. It is the electronic exchange of information using a computer network. E-mails tend to be asynchronous (that is,

FIGURE 5.9. **E-mail best practices**

1. Encrypt during transmission.
2. Avoid group e-mails that could compromise confidentiality. If group e-mails are sent, the blind copy function should be used.
3. Confirm the e-mail address of the patient being communicated with to avoid errant e-mails and to avoid responding to e-mails that may have been sent by someone else (under the guise of the patient's identity).
4. Use e-mail addresses that have been stored in memory. Routinely verify their continued validity.
5. Avoid answering e-mails from an unsecured location, as this may compromise security.
6. Be cautious about opening e-mail attachments that could contain viruses.
7. Train staff on e-mail policies and procedures.

Source: Rinehart-Thompson 2011

the parties communicate at different times) and readily allow a sender to distribute one message to multiple people. Due to the federal e-discovery rules, e-mails are discoverable in federal courts and in states where the rules have been adopted. In addition to the risk of being subject to discovery, e-mails also present privacy and security risks that accompany data transmission. Figure 5.9 lists best practices for minimizing privacy and security breaches associated with e-mails. If a covered entity, business associate, or subcontractor commits a breach, it must follow HIPAA breach notification requirements.

Text Messaging

Text messaging is also used in healthcare. It is the electronic exchange of information between mobile electronic devices using a telephone network. Text messages tend to be more synchronous, and thus more immediate, than e-mailing because of their brevity and immediate display on device screens. It can be used for provider-to-provider communication as well as provider-to-patient communication. For example, it can be used to remind patients to take their medications. It also presents privacy and security risks. Figure 5.10 lists best practices for minimizing privacy and security breaches associated with text messaging. If a covered entity, business associate, or subcontractor commits a breach, it must follow HIPAA breach notification requirements.

Facsimiles

A **facsimile (fax)** is an electronic transmission of paper or electronic information via telephone lines to an identified location. A facsimile (fax) machine is used to carry out this transmission. As with any electronic transmission, its efficiency may be outweighed by privacy and security risks. These include sending health information to the wrong recipient, or finding that it has been intercepted in transit or after it has reached its destination. Faxed information must be protected. Figure 5.11 lists best practices for minimizing privacy and security breaches associated with facsimiles. If a covered entity, business associate, or subcontractor commits a breach, it must follow HIPAA breach notification requirements.

FIGURE 5.10. Text messaging best practices

1. Encrypt during transmission.
2. Avoid text messages to more than one patient that could compromise confidentiality.
3. Confirm the telephone number of the patient being communicated with to avoid errant text messages and to avoid responding to text messages that may have been sent by someone else (under the guise of the patient's identity).
4. Use telephone numbers that have been stored in memory. Routinely verify their continued validity.
5. Train staff on text messaging policies and procedures.

Source: Rinehart-Thompson 2011

FIGURE 5.11. Facsimile best practices

1. Place fax machines in secure locations.
2. Include confidentiality cover sheets when transmitting information via fax, including the name and contact information of the intended recipient. The sheet should also tell recipients who to contact if information has been received in error and advise them to destroy the information.
3. Confirm fax numbers before sending information.
4. Pre-program frequently used fax numbers to avoid misdialed numbers. Routinely verify the pre-programmed numbers.
5. Provide for encryption during transit.
6. Fax information only when it is necessary to do so (for example, urgent medical situations).
7. Avoid faxing highly sensitive information (for example, behavioral health, HIV/AIDS, substance abuse, and genetic information).
8. Train staff on fax policies and procedures.

Source: Rinehart-Thompson 2011

Telemedicine

Telemedicine involves electronic communication to exchange medical information with the ultimate goal of improving patient health. It is a broad term that encompasses many activities including continuing medical education, remote monitoring of patient vital signs, and transmission of radiologic images for review and interpretation. As some of these activities indicate, telemedicine often links patients and providers so that face-to-face interaction is not necessary. This is particularly helpful where patients live in remote areas and travel is difficult for both the patient and the provider. Some of the technologies described in the previous sections, such as e-mails and text messaging, can also be considered telemedicine if they are used to improve patient health. If telemedicine includes these technologies, best practices for those technologies should be used. Data should be encrypted to protect the privacy and security of patient information. If a covered entity, business associate, or subcontractor commits a breach, it must follow HIPAA breach notification requirements.

CHECK YOUR UNDERSTANDING 5.2

Instructions: Indicate whether the following statements are true or false (T or F).

1. A disaster recovery plan restores critical services as quickly as possible after an event.
2. An emergency mode of operations includes identifying the minimum number of people needed to complete each function.
3. Data recovery should not include obtaining copies of records from entities that received records from the organization.
4. Health information exchange (HIE) opt-out models are prohibited by the HIPAA Security Rule.
5. A patient portal is often hosted and controlled by a provider or payer.

REAL-WORLD CASE

In August 2005, the Gulf Coast was struck by one of the most severe natural disasters the country has experienced. In New Orleans, the devastation caused by Hurricane Katrina was heightened when the city's levee system failed. Following are the experiences of one New Orleans hospital that had to test its disaster plan and learned from that experience.

Chalmette Medical Center is a 250-bed, two-story facility in New Orleans, Louisiana, part of Universal Health Services (UHS), Inc., headquartered in King of Prussia, Pennsylvania. The legal health record was hybrid, containing both electronic and paper documentation. The data center is located in Pennsylvania.

As the storm formed, the facility's first priority was the patients. If they could be discharged, they were. If they could not, their emergency contact information was confirmed. Staff then began to secure the physical facility and obtain additional needed supplies such as food and fuel for generators. Communication was critical, so it was confirmed that all key team members had mobile communication devices. Additionally, routine status meetings were held. Patient records were placed in rooms with the patients (with electronic information printed) so their health information would be with them if they had to be evacuated.

When the storm made landfall, electricity and cell phone coverage was disrupted. Staff and patients remained in the facility. Evacuation was not an option because of the lack of ambulances and gridlock on the roads. Initial relief at the storm's passing was short-lived as the levee system failed and the city was flooded. Evacuation then became absolutely necessary, with the most acute patients evacuated first via roof-top helicopter. Due to power outages, family notification was not possible.

The UHS headquarters in Pennsylvania created a command center to manager critical communications. Facility data repositories were used to obtain patient and employee information. They were then copied into working databases to track individuals' locations and telephone inquiries. A toll-free number was created to provide information to callers, including information about the patient evacuation and the location of employees. Release of information requests were also facilitated as a release-of-information database was constructed to track and verify requests and share online information. Fortunately, the electronic portion of patients' health records were stored in a remote data center and could be accessed. In the days that followed, UHS created a database to track incoming donations and funds dispensed for displaced employees.

Chalmette Medical Center had to be closed as it remained underwater for a significant period and experienced severe structural damage. A tax levy was passed to reopen the facility, with a revision to the bed size and services provided. Lessons were learned from the Hurricane Katrina experience, such as:

- Advance disaster planning is essential.
- Disaster plans must be flexible.
- An organization cannot have too much communication, either verbal or written. All tools must be considered as cell phones provide no value if cell towers are down. In that case, satellite phones become critical.
- Gasoline is needed to run generators.
- A good staffing plan must be in place to meet patients' needs and not to burn out staff.
- People will step up to the plate when they are needed.
- A command center may become necessary; know how to create and operate one.
- Shelters should accommodate chronic conditions, with emergency rooms reserved for acutely ill patients.
- Electronic records located remotely can save patients' lives.
- Personal health records are important in treating patients during disaster recovery. (Reino and Hyde 2006)

SUMMARY

In anticipation of threats that can disrupt operations, it is important for an organization to perform risk analysis and risk management activities. These are also required by the HIPAA Security Rule. There are many steps involved in conducting a risk analysis; one of the most important is to identify threats, which can be categorized as internal and external to the organization or as those created by humans versus those created by natural and environmental factors. A specific type of human threat is identity theft, which has financial consequences for the victim, and medical identity theft, which is a type of identity theft that has both financial and medical consequences. Because of the prevalence of identity theft, the Federal Trade Commission issued the Red Flags Rule.

If a threat becomes a reality, it is important for an organization to have a contingency plan in place, focusing on disaster recovery, business continuity, and emergency mode of operations. For the health information manager, an important part of these activities is the management and recovery of patient data.

This chapter discussed the importance of anticipating threats and having a plan to respond to threats that become actual events. Additionally, it is important to address the privacy and security of health information used in HIEs and transmitted by ubiquitous communication methods such as e-mails and text messaging.

REFERENCES

Amatayakul, M. 2012. *Electronic Health Records: A Practical Guide for Professionals and Organizations,* 5th ed. Chicago: AHIMA.

American Health Information Management Association. 2012a. *Pocket Glossary for Health Information Management and Technology*, 3rd ed. Chicago: AHIMA.

American Health Information Management Association. 2012b. The 10 security domains (updated). *Journal of AHIMA* 83(5): 48–52. http://library.ahima.org/xpedio/groups/public/documents/ahima/bok1_049602.hcsp?dDocName=bok1_049602.

American Health Information Management Association. 2011. HIE Management and Operational Considerations. *Journal of AHIMA* 82(5): 56–61.

American Health Information Management Association. 2010a. Disaster Planning for Health Information (Updated). http://library.ahima.org/xpedio/groups/public/documents/ahima/bok1_048638.hcsp?dDocName=bok1_048638.

American Health Information Management Association. 2010b. Health Information Exchange (HIE) Consumer Brochure. http://library.ahima.org/xpedio/groups/public/documents/ahima/bok1_048939.pdf.

American Recovery and Reinvestment Act of 2009. Title XIII: Health Information Technology, Subtitle D: Privacy, Part 1: Improved Privacy Provisions and Security Provisions, Sections 13402.

Department of Health and Human Services. 2012. Health Information Privacy. Breaches Affecting 500 or More Individuals. http://www.hhs.gov/ocr/privacy/hipaa/administrative/breachnotificationrule/breachtool.html.

Dixon, P. 2006. Medical identity theft: The information crime that can kill you. World Privacy Forum. http://www.worldprivacyforum.org/medicalidentitytheft.html.

Federal Trade Commission. Fighting Fraud With the Red Flags Rule. n.d. http://www.ftc.gov/bcp/edu/microsites/redflagsrule/index.shtml.

Federal Trade Commission. 2007. Identity Theft Red Flags and Address Discrepancies Under the Fair and Accurate Credit Transaction Act of 20003. 16 CFR Part 681. *Federal Register* 72(217): 63718-63775.

Gellman, R., and P. Dixon. 2009. Red Flag and address discrepancy requirements: Suggestions for health care providers. Version 2. Cardiff by the Sea, CA: World Privacy Forum.

Halpert, A.M. 2008a. Complying with the Privacy Rule during a Disaster—Part 1: An Overview of Plan Development, Data Backup, and Recovery. *Journal of AHIMA* 79(4): 60–61. http://library.ahima.org/xpedio/groups/public/documents/ahima/bok1_037471.hcsp?dDocName=bok1_037471.

Halpert, A.M. 2008b. Complying with the Privacy Rule during a Disaster—Part 2. *Journal of AHIMA* 79(5): 58–59. http://library.ahima.org/xpedio/groups/public/documents/ahima/bok1_038096 .hcsp?dDocName=bok1_038096.

LaTour, K. and S. Eichenwald-Maki (eds.) 2010. *Health Information Management: Concepts, Principles, and Practice.* 3rd ed. Chicago: AHIMA.

National Institute of Standards and Technology. 2002. *Risk Management Guide for Information Technology Systems.* http://csrc.nist.gov/publications/nistpubs/800-30/sp800-30.pdf.

Office of the National Coordinator for Health Information Technology. US Department of Health and Human Services. 2008. Nationwide Privacy and Security Framework For Electronic Exchange of Individually Identifiable Health Information. http://healthit.hhs.gov/portal/server.pt?open=512&mode =2&cached=true&objID=1173.

Reino, L. and C. Hyde. 2006. Disaster recovery: The importance in managing information in the wake of Hurricane Katrina. *AHIMA's 78th National Convention and Exhibit Proceedings.*

Rinehart-Thompson, L. 2011. AHIMA E-Learning Exam Prep Course: CHPS Domain 3—Information Technology/Physical and Technical Safeguards.

Walsh, T. 2011. AHIMA practice brief: Security risk analysis and management: An overview (updated). http://library.ahima.org/xpedio/groups/public/documents/ahima/bok1_048622 .hcsp?dDocName=bok1_048622

Warner, D. 2011 (May). HIE patient consent model options. *Journal of AHIMA* 82(5): 48–49. http://library.ahima.org/xpedio/groups/secure/documents/ahima/bok1_048929 .hcsp?dDocName=bok1_048929.

45 CFR 164.308(a)(1)(ii)(A): Risk Analysis. 2006.

45 CFR 164.308(a)(1)(ii)(B): Risk Management. 2006.

45 CFR 164.308(a)(7)(ii)(A): Data Backup Plan. 2006.

CHAPTER **6**

Key Changes under HITECH

Learning Objectives

- Describe the federal rulemaking process and types of rules

- Explain the HITECH changes as they affect business associates and subcontractors

- Define a breach of protected health information and describe HITECH's breach notification requirements

- Identify the HIPAA individual rights that are affected by HITECH

- Compare proposed changes to the accounting of disclosures requirement with the proposed access report

- Describe changes to the minimum necessary requirement per HITECH

- Explain how HITECH affects personal health record vendors

- Identify HITECH's changes to marketing, fundraising, and the sale of information

- Describe changes to enforcement and penalties under HITECH

- Explain how HITECH changes the status of decedents' protected health information

- Identify HITECH's changes to research authorization requirements

- Describe how HITECH impacts student immunization records

- Compare previous Notice of Privacy Practices content requirements with new requirements under HITECH

- Compare changes set forth in HITECH (February 2009) with those in the January 2013 final rule

KEY TERMS

Access

Access report

Accounting of disclosures

Administrative Procedure Act (APA)

American Recovery and Reinvestment Act (ARRA)

Breach

Breach notification

Business associate (BA)

Business associate agreement (BAA)

Code of Federal Regulations (CFR)

Covered entity

Direct final rule

Enforcement Rule

Federal Register

Final rule

Formal rulemaking

Fundraising

Genetic Information and Nondiscrimination Act (GINA) of 2008

Government Accountability Office (GAO)

Harm threshold

Health Information Technology for Economic and Clinical Health (HITECH) Act

Informal rulemaking

Interim final rule

Major rule

Marketing

Minimum necessary

Notice of Privacy Practices (NPP)

Notice of Proposed Rulemaking (NPRM)

Office for Civil Rights (OCR)

Office of Management and Budget (OMB)

Parens patriae

Personal health record vendor

Promulgation

Proposed rule

Protected health information (PHI)

Restriction request

Sale of information

Subcontractor

Tiered penalties

United States Department of Health and Human Services (HHS)

INTRODUCTION

As described in earlier chapters, the HIPAA statute was passed in 1996 and implemented in 2003 and 2005 for privacy and security, respectively. However, the **Health Information Technology for Economic and Clinical Health (HITECH) Act** of the **American Recovery and Reinvestment Act (ARRA)**, which was signed into law on February 17, 2009, made significant changes to HIPAA. This chapter will discuss HITECH provisions that impact HIPAA. The compliance date for these provisions was initially set at February 17, 2010, one year after the law was signed. However, interim final rules relating to breach notification and enforcement were also published in 2009, and proposed rules were published in 2010 and 2011. In January 2013, a final rule was published that encompasses provisions in both of the interim final rules and the 2010 proposed rule. It affirms HITECH's privacy, security, enforcement, and breach notification requirements. By expanding individuals' rights and imposing greater obligations on both covered entities and business associates, HITECH promises to be a challenge for those required to comply with it.

Section 1: Overview of Federal Rulemaking Process

Once a statute is passed by Congress and signed by the president, authority may be given to an administrative agency to write the rules (administrative laws) that implement the statute. For HIPAA, this authority is given to the **United States Department of Health and Human Services (HHS)**. HHS is the cabinet-level federal agency that oversees all the health- and human-services–related activities of the federal government and administers federal regulations (AHIMA 2012). However, HHS authority is not without limitations. The **Administrative Procedure Act (APA)** (5 USC § 551 et seq.) imposes procedural uniformity on federal agencies and governs how federal administrative agencies may propose and establish rules (also referred to as regulations) that serve to fill in the details of a statute. The APA was created in 1946 in response to concerns about the level of power that the many federal agencies newly created under President Roosevelt's post-Depression New Deal would have.

Types of Rulemaking

There are two main categories of rulemaking: formal and informal. **Formal rulemaking** is one way that a federal administrative agency creates an administrative rule. According to the APA, if formal rulemaking is required, a rule cannot be implemented unless the applicable agency has previously conducted a hearing that adheres to a trial format. Its use in federal rulemaking is limited, applying to rules such as those that establish utility rates (Copeland 2011). The rulemaking process that affects HIPAA rules is informal rulemaking. **Informal rulemaking** is another way that a federal administrative agency creates an administrative rule. According to the APA, where informal rulemaking applies, a rule must be published so that interested parties can utilize a notice and comment period to respond to the published rule. After comments are received, they are analyzed and responded to and a final rule is prepared and published. There is a waiting period, which varies based on the federal agency and the nature of the rule, before the final rule is effective (Copeland 2011). The notice and comment period inherent to informal rulemaking is particularly important because it allows individuals and organizations affected by the rule to provide input. Interested parties must be given an adequate amount of time to review the rule and to comment. **Promulgation** is the formal declaration of an administrative law.

Proposed Rules

A **proposed rule** is the first draft of an administrative rule. It may be either a new rule or a proposed change to an existing rule. Publication of the proposed rule in the *Federal Register* as a notice calling for public comment is called a **notice of proposed rulemaking (NPRM)**. An NPRM must offer an opportunity to the public at large—including interested individuals or organizations—to submit comments within a specified time period (AHIMA 2012). However, a proposed rule is not always required. A rule may first be published as one of the various types of final rules.

Types of Final Rules

There are three types of final rules: interim final rules, direct final rules, and final rules. Each of these will be briefly discussed.

Interim Final Rule

An **interim final rule** is published without being preceded by an NPRM (Copeland 2011). It is a final rule that has the full force and effect of law; however, it must offer a post-promulgation opportunity for public comments. Based on public comments received, the federal agency may issue a revised final rule or it may confirm the interim final rule as the final rule that will continue to be effective.

Direct Final Rule

A **direct final rule** is also published without being preceded by an NPRM. It is published with a statement that the rule is set to become effective on an established date unless adverse comments are received within a specified timeframe. The federal agency has a duty to withdraw the rule if adverse comments are received and it may then publish the rule as a proposed rule (Copeland 2011). If adverse comments are not received, however, it remains as a final rule. This mechanism is generally used for noncontroversial rules.

Final Rule

A **final rule** is published after public comments are considered in response to a proposed rule. Alternatively, as discussed previously, an interim final rule or direct final rule may become the final rule. Generally, the APA specifies that a final rule cannot become effective for at least 30 days after publication (Copeland 2011).

Governmental Oversight

Most final rules must be submitted to Congress and the **Government Accountability Office (GAO)**, an independent agency that works on behalf of Congress to audit how the federal government spends taxpayer dollars, before the final rules can take effect. If a rule is considered a **major rule**, which is estimated to cost over $100 million, it must also be submitted to the **Office of Management and Budget (OMB)** for analysis (Copeland 2011). The OMB reviews rules for consistency with presidential policies and budgetary priorities. Submission of a rule to the OMB is a process that is carefully watched and eagerly anticipated by interested parties. This is because it is a final step that indicates the rule is close to being released. The OMB has 90 days to review a rule, but it may extend its review up to 120 days or even longer if it obtains agreement from the director of the agency that created the rule.

The *Federal Register*

The *Federal Register* is a daily publication of the US Government Printing Office that reports all changes in regulations (AHIMA 2012). The APA requires that federal agencies publish proposed new rules, proposed changes to rules, and final rules in the *Federal Register* so they are available to the public (Copeland 2011). After a final rule is published in the *Federal Register*, it then must be placed in the **Code of Federal Regulations (CFR)**, the permanent location of administrative laws.

Section 2: HITECH Privacy Provisions

HITECH's privacy and security provisions are located in Title XIII (Health Information Technology), Subtitle D (Privacy), Part I (Improved Privacy Provisions and Security Provisions). These provisions encompass sections 13401 through 13411. Additionally, Section 13400 sets forth applicable definitions. These are part of the statute that was signed into law on February 17, 2009. Figure 6.1 sequentially outlines the content of each of the sections, along with the corresponding section numbers. Two interim final rules relating to breach notification and enforcement (to update a pre-HITECH 2006 final enforcement rule) were published by the Department of Health and Human Services on August 24, 2009 and October 30, 2009. Some of the provisions that will be discussed were not part of the original HITECH legislation. Instead, they first appeared as proposed rules in subsequent Notices of Proposed Rulemaking on July 14, 2010 and May 31, 2011. These are denoted in figures 6.1 and 6.2. The January 2013 final rule, "Modifications to the HIPAA Privacy, Security, Enforcement, and Breach Notification Rules," was published in the *Federal Register* on January 25, 2013. It finalizes the two interim final rules (AHIMA 2013). It also finalizes provisions first introduced in the July 2010 proposed rule, but it does not address the access report (related to the Accounting of Disclosures provision), which was first introduced in the May 2011 proposed rule. Thus, the Accounting of Disclosures provisions remain outstanding, to be released at a later date. The January 2013 final rule also adds HIPAA requirements related to the **Genetic Information Nondiscrimination Act (GINA) of 2008**. The rule defines genetic information as health information and sets forth rules relative to genetic information a health plan may or may not use for underwriting and other activities (AHIMA 2013). The final rule is effective March 26, 2013 with a compliance date of September 23, 2013, although there are varying compliance deadlines for business associate agreements depending on whether or not they are currently compliant with HIPAA (AHIMA 2013). This chapter reflects provisions of the January 2013 final rule relative to HIPAA.

FIGURE 6.1.	HITECH privacy provisions (sequential, by section number)
13400	Definitions
13401	BAs (security/penalties)
13402	Breach notification
13403	Regional privacy officers/education initiative (not discussed in this chapter)
13404	BAs (privacy/penalties)
13405	Access
	Restriction requests
	Accounting of disclosures
	Minimum necessary
	Sale of information

(Continued on next page)

FIGURE 6.1.	(Continued)
13406	Marketing
	Fundraising
13407	PHR vendors
13408	BAs (HIEs, RHIOs, e-prescribing gateways, PHR vendors, PSOs)
13409	Enforcement and penalties: criminal penalties (individuals)
13410	Enforcement and penalties: tiers
	Enforcement and penalties: state Attorneys General
	Enforcement and penalties: individual compensation
13411	Enforcement and penalties: audits
NPRMs:	PHI of decedents (7/14/10 NPRM)
	Research authorization requirements (7/14/10 NPRM)
	Student immunization records (7/14/10 NPRM)
	Notice of privacy practices (7/14/10 AND 5/31/11 NPRM)
	Access report (5/31/11 NPRM)

FIGURE 6.2.	HITECH provisions, by date first introduced				
Provision	HITECH	2/09 HITECH	7/10 NPRM	5/11 NPRM
BAs and subcontractors	13401	X		
	13404			
	13408			
Breach notification	13402	X		
Access	13405	X		
Restriction requests	13405	X		
Accounting of disclosures	13405	X		
Access report				X
Minimum necessary	13405	X		
Personal health record vendors	13407	X		
Marketing	13406	X		
Fundraising	13406	X		
Sale of information	13405	X		

FIGURE 6.2. (Continued)				
Provision	HITECH	2/09 HITECH	7/10 NPRM	5/11 NPRM
Attorneys General	13410	X		
Audits	13411	X		
Individual prosecution	13409	X		
Tiered penalties	13410	X		
Individual compensation	13410	X		
PHI of decedents			X	
Research authorization requirements			X	
Student immunization records			X	
Notice of privacy practices			X	X

Major revisions to HIPAA include changes to requirements relating to business associates and subcontractors; breach notification; individual rights (namely access, restriction requests, accounting of disclosures, and access report); minimum necessary; personal health record vendors; marketing; fundraising; sale of information; increased enforcement and penalties for noncompliance; **protected health information (PHI)** of decedents; research authorization requirements; student immunization records; and changes to the notice of privacy practices.

Business Associates and Subcontractors (Sections 13401, 13404, 13408)

One of the most significant changes under HITECH is the increased inclusion and visibility of **business associates (BAs)**. HIPAA regulations now apply to BAs for the first time, and this includes increased exposure to liability. Under HITECH, responsibilities and liabilities previously assumed by covered entities only for wrongful uses and disclosures are now generally applied to BAs, as well. It is now much riskier for an organization or individual to become a BA.

First, BAs are now obligated by law to comply with HIPAA, not by contract alone. What this means is that it is now the nature of the relationship—not the contract—that makes a person or an organization a BA. People or entities that meet the definition of business associate, even if they have not entered into a **business associate agreement (BAA)** with a **covered entity**, must fulfill requirements imposed on BAs (AHIMA 2009). The following example provides clarification: prior to HITECH, a medical transcriptionist who transcribed reports for a physician's office met the definition of a BA (that is, he used PHI on behalf of the covered entity). However, if the physician's office failed to initiate a BAA with the transcriptionist, the transcriptionist was not bound to comply with HIPAA because the transcriptionist was not identified as a BA by contract. Under HITECH, however, the nature of the transcriptionist's work and his relationship with the physician's office (that is, using PHI on behalf of a covered entity) automatically makes the transcriptionist a BA (by law), even if no BAA is in place.

In addition to expanding the scope of those who are BAs, even without a contract or BAA, HITECH now specifically includes the following as BAs: patient safety organizations (PSOs), which receive information in order to analyze patient safety issues; health information exchanges (HIEs) and health information organizations which electronically share health information among providers; e-prescribing gateways, which serve as intermediaries between prescribing physicians and pharmacies; other persons who facilitate data transmissions; and **personal health record (PHR) vendors** that, by contract, enable covered entities to offer PHRs to their patient as part of the covered entity's electronic health record (ARRA 2009; AHIMA 2010).

HITECH also specifically includes a BA's **subcontractors**, naming them as BAs under HIPAA if they require access to an individual's PHI (AHIMA 2010). Once again, it does not matter whether a BAA has been signed. If a person or organization meets the definition of a subcontractor, it is bound by HIPAA. Nonetheless, BAs do have an obligation to initiate BAAs with their subcontractors and obtain satisfactory assurance from them that they meet the requirements of the BAA. Each subsequent subcontractor, in turn, must follow the same process with their own subcontractors (AHIMA 2013). With the expanded applicability of BAs and their subcontractors, it is important that BAs, whether direct BAs of the covered entity or subsequent subcontractors, train their workforce on HIPAA compliance and ensure their subcontractors do the same, as they all can be held liable for violating HIPAA (AHIMA 2013).

Organizations or individuals that meet the definition of BA (and are BAs by law) must now comply with certain provisions of HIPAA. These include breach notification, accounting of disclosures and restrictions on the sale of health information (all of which are discussed later in this chapter). HIPAA's Security Rule also now applies broadly to BAs. BAs must comply with the administrative, physical, and technical safeguards of the HIPAA Security Rule. The HIPAA Security Rule also imposes policy and procedure requirements, as well as documentation requirements, which BAs must comply with as well (AHIMA 2009). A BA obligation to comply with the Security Rule is to be incorporated into the BAA. (The requirements of the HIPAA Security Rule are discussed in chapter 4.) BAs are also subject to the same civil and criminal penalties that covered entities face for violating either the Privacy or Security Rule (AHIMA 2009).

Greater responsibility for HIPAA compliance has now shifted so that covered entities are no longer the primary gatekeepers. In many respects, BAs are held equally responsible. Covered entities were historically required to respond to BA noncompliance, but BAs are now also required (per HITECH) to respond to covered entity noncompliance by requiring corrective action or severing the relationship with the covered entity.

Breach Notification (Section 13402)

Under HIPAA as originally implemented, the wrongful use or disclosure of an individual's PHI required a covered entity to mitigate, or lessen the harmful effect, as much as possible. However, the covered entity had discretion in deciding whether mitigation included notifying the individual of the breach or not. This discretion has been taken away under HITECH through the addition of **breach notification** requirements. HITECH's breach notification requirements were published in the August 2009 interim final rule. The January 2013 final rule replaced the August 2009 interim final rule's "harm threshold" and replaced it with a more objective standard (AHIMA 2013). HITECH's requirements are significant because they require both covered entities and BAs to conduct breach notifications. Subcontractors must report breaches to the BA that holds its contract. In turn, the BA must notify the covered entity, who must notify affected individuals (AHIMA 2013). Breach notification requirements place both covered entities and BAs on regulatory agencies' radars. They also place organizations in the media spotlight when PHI is handled inappropriately. It is undesirable to an organization to be featured on the Internet, in the newspaper, or on the evening news for mishandling PHI.

What Is a Breach?

HITECH defines a **breach** as an "unauthorized acquisition, access, use, or disclosure of PHI which compromises the security or privacy of such information" (ARRA 2009). Not every situation that fits the definition is a breach, however. HITECH includes exceptions to the breach definition, and these are outlined in figure 6.3.

FIGURE 6.3.	Exceptions to the definition of breach
Unintentional acquisition	Breach does not include any unintentional acquisition, access, or use of PHI by a workforce member acting under the authority of a covered entity or BA, and made in good faith and within the scope of authority (information cannot be further used or disclosed in impermissible manner) Example: A staff member in the Quality Improvement Department intended to send an e-mail containing PHI to her colleague, Jane Smith, in the same department. She accidentally selected the e-mail address of Jay Smith, an employee in the Respiratory Therapy Department. Jay Smith opened the e-mail but deleted it immediately without reading it when he saw that it was intended for Jane Smith.
Inadvertent disclosure	Breach does not include any inadvertent disclosure of PHI from a person authorized to access PHI at a covered entity or BA to another person authorized to access PHI at the covered entity or BA, or organized healthcare arrangement in which the covered entity participates (information cannot be further used or disclosed in impermissible manner) Example: A dietician has completed a nutrition care plan for Albert Jones. She hands the information to Mary Clark, a nurse on Mr. Jones' unit. However, Mary is not Mr. Jones' nurse. Cindy Lee is. Cindy, without looking at its contents, either gives the information to Mary or places it in Mr. Jones' chart.
Recipient would not have been able to retain information	Breach does not include disclosure of PHI if the covered entity or BA has a good faith belief the unauthorized individual who received the PHI would not be able to retain the information Example: Timmy's mother had requested a copy of Timmy's recent test results from his pediatrician's office. She went into the office to pick them up but they were not immediately available. While she waited in the waiting room, Denise, an office assistant, brought the test results out and handed them to another mother. As soon as she handed the results to the other mother, Denise realized her mistake. She took them back immediately, apologized to both parties, and gave the results to Timmy's mother.

Source: ARRA 2009; HHS 2009

Breach notification requirements apply only to unsecured PHI, which is PHI that has not been made "unusable, unreadable, or indecipherable to unauthorized persons through the use of technology or methodology specified by the Secretary in guidance" (AHIMA 2013). Thus, the loss or theft of data that has been secured (such as by encryption) is not a breach. As noted above, a breach is an act that "compromises security or privacy." The August 2009 interim final rule interpreted this to mean that it "poses a significant risk of financial, reputational, or other harm to the individual" (HHS 2009). One of the dilemmas surrounding breach identification was the burden that HITECH (as set forth in the August 2009 interim final rule) placed on covered entities and BAs to determine whether or not a particular incident fit this "**harm threshold**" by posing a significant risk of harm to the individual(s) whose information was breached. Many organizations were not comfortable making this determination and facing the possibility of being penalized for interpreting the level of harm incorrectly (particularly if a determination is made that an incident did not meet the harm threshold). The January 2013 final rule removed the harm threshold and clarified the definition of breach in a more objective way. Now, "an impermissible use or disclosure of PHI is presumed to be a breach unless the covered entity or BA demonstrates that there is a low probability that the PHI has been compromised" (AHIMA 2013).

Notification

Covered entities and BAs are subject to HHS-issued breach notification regulations. Noncovered entities and non-BAs are subject to companion breach notification regulations. Per the 2013 final rule, breach notification is required unless a covered entity or BA demonstrates through a risk assessment that the probability of the PHI having been compromised is low. (This replaces the previous subjective "significant risk of harm to the individual" standard.) The risk assessment must consider at least the following:

1. Nature and extent of PHI involved (including identifier types);
2. The unauthorized person(s) the disclosure was made to, or who used the PHI (and whether the person has an obligation to protect the PHI);
3. Whether or not the PHI was actually acquired or viewed by the unauthorized person(s), versus whether an opportunity merely existed; and
4. The extent to which the covered entity or BA has mitigated the risk to the PHI.

The final rule specifies that risk assessments must also be conducted in response to impermissible uses and disclosures of limited data sets. (AHIMA 2013)

Breaches are treated as discovered when the breach is first known or should reasonably have been known. Individuals whose information has been breached must be notified without unreasonable delay (no more than 60 days), by first-class mail. The covered entity may provide notification through a faster method (such as telephone) if there is the potential for "imminent misuse." Figure 6.4 shows the information that must be provided to individuals whose PHI has been breached.

If more than nine individuals are affected and written notice is unsuccessful, notification through web postings and use of the media are recommended. Five hundred is a significant number with regard to breach notification. If 500 or more people are affected by a breach, the Secretary of HHS must be notified immediately. Prominent media outlets must be contacted if the number of affected individuals per state reaches 500 or more. For example, if a breach of PHI affecting 800 individuals includes 300 individuals residing in Ohio; 250 individuals residing in Michigan; and 250 individuals residing in Pennsylvania, media outlets would not have to be notified because the total did not reach 500 in any one state (AHIMA 2013). This exception does not apply to notifications to HHS.

Substitute notices (for example, on the covered entity's website) should be provided if the covered entity has insufficient or outdated contact information for the affected individuals. A covered entity is ultimately responsible to notify individuals affected by its BA's breaches, but the covered entity has discretion to delegate that responsibility to the BA (AHIMA 2013).

FIGURE 6.4.	Information shared with individuals whose PHI has been breached
A description of what occurred (including date of breach and date that breach was discovered)	
The types of unsecured PHI that were involved (such as name, social security number, date of birth, home address, and account number)	
Steps that the individual may take to protect himself or herself	
What the entity is doing to investigate, mitigate, and prevent future occurrences	
Contact information for the individual to ask questions and receive updates	

Source: AHIMA 2009; ARRA 2009

Breach Report

Regardless of the size of a breach, all breaches must be reported to HHS. HHS maintains an online breach reporting system. Breaches involving fewer than 500 individuals may be logged internally on a case-by-case basis, but all breaches must have been entered into the HHS system and submitted annually (thus, reported to HHS) no more than 60 days after the end of the calendar year when the breaches were discovered.

If a breach involves 500 or more individuals, it must be reported to HHS immediately. Thereafter, the breach is posted on the HHS website (HHS 2012). By December 2012, over 510 breaches involving 500 or more individuals and totaling over 19 million records had been reported and posted (HHS 2012). The number of individuals affected ranged from 500 upward to 4,901,432 in a September 2011 breach involving the loss of backup tapes by Tricare Management Activity in Virginia. Breaches include theft, loss, unauthorized access and disclosure, hacking, and improper disposal. Portable devices such as laptop computers present one of the greatest breach risks, although breaches of portable devices have involved both malicious (for example, theft) and accidental (for example, loss) activities. The HHS database of breaches may be searched by name of covered entity, state, number of individuals affected, date of breach, type of breach, and location of breached information (such as paper, laptop computer, or network server).

CHECK YOUR UNDERSTANDING 6.1

Instructions: Indicate whether the following statements are true or false (T or F).

1. All types of final administrative rules must be preceded by a Notice of Proposed Rulemaking.
2. A BA must only comply with HIPAA if a written contract is in place that identifies it as a BA.
3. The theft of data that has been secured does not constitute a breach.
4. If 500 or more people are affected by a PHI breach, the Secretary of HHS must be notified immediately.
5. Per HITECH, BAs must comply with the administrative, physical, and technical safeguards of the HIPAA Security Rule

Individual Rights (Section 13405)

Three of the five individual rights that HIPAA provides have been affected by HITECH. These include access, restriction requests, and accounting of disclosures. Additionally, the access report is a proposed individual right that is intertwined with the accounting of disclosures.

Access (Section 13405)

As discussed in chapter 3, HIPAA gives an individual the right to **access** their own PHI. This includes inspecting and obtaining a copy of PHI contained in a designated record set (DRS) and transmitting PHI to third parties upon the individual's request. HITECH has revised this right by requiring covered entities with EHRs to make PHI available electronically if the individual requests it, in the format requested if it is readily producible. Additionally, upon individual request, covered entities are to transmit PHI electronically to a person or entity that the individual has designated. When a covered entity transmits PHI electronically, it must ensure that reasonable safeguards are in place. This includes warning the individual of the risk of sending PHI via unencrypted e-mail. If the individual still desires to have PHI transmitted in this manner, however, the covered entity must comply with the individual's wishes.

Requirements regarding fees have not changed under HITECH. They are still permitted as long as they do not exceed the labor (including compiling or scanning records or burning disks), supplies, and postage associated with providing the information (AHIMA 2013). This limitation is consistent with previous HIPAA requirements and supersedes state laws that permit fees above an organization's actual costs. The January 2013 final rule clarifies that retrieval fees are not allowed, regardless of whether they are standard fees or based on actual retrieval costs (AHIMA 2013).

Restriction Requests (Section 13405)

HIPAA has required that an individual be permitted to make a **restriction request** (that is, an individual may ask a covered entity to restrict the uses and disclosures of PHI for carrying out treatment, payment, and healthcare operations [TPO]). As originally written, covered entities only had to consider the requests; they did not have to agree to them.

HITECH has implemented one important exception to this provision. Under HITECH, a covered entity must comply with an individual's request, unless otherwise required by law, if a disclosure would be made to a health plan for payment or healthcare operations (and not for treatment) and the PHI pertains solely to an item or service that has been paid for in full other than by the health plan (AHIMA 2009 and AHIMA 2013). The logistics of carrying out this requirement, however, will be complex, particularly where future disclosures are involved. Covered entities must take care to ensure that restricted PHI is not inadvertently disclosed, in violation of the restriction, with subsequent legitimate disclosures.

Accounting of Disclosures (Section 13405)

The **accounting of disclosures** has likely been the most controversial individual right since HIPAA's implementation in 2003. Administratively burdensome and infrequently used by individuals, there was discussion that perhaps this individual right would be retired. On the contrary, HITECH has added to the right.

Per HITECH, covered entities using or maintaining an EHR would be required to include TPO disclosures in their accounting of disclosures (TPO was an exception under HIPAA as originally drafted). HITECH's compliance timetable would depend on when covered entities acquired their EHRs. The compliance dates for covered entities with more recent EHR acquisitions would occur sooner, presumably because the newer systems would better be able to handle the increased volume and more complex requirements than older systems could. HITECH did, however, shorten the time frame for an accounting of disclosures. Previously, an accounting had to include disclosures made during the previous six years. This has been shortened to disclosures made during the previous three years (AHIMA 2009). For covered entities without an EHR, TPO continues to be a significant exception to the accounting of disclosures requirement under HITECH. Additionally, under HITECH BAs must respond to accounting requests made directly to them (AHIMA 2009). This provision was not addressed in the January 2013 final rule. A rule addressing the accounting of disclosures and associated access report (discussed below) is expected to be released at a future date.

Access Report (May 31, 2011 NPRM)

Note: Although this provision did not first appear until the May 31, 2011 NPRM was published, it is discussed here because it is a proposed individual right that is intertwined with the accounting of disclosures individual right.

As covered entities and BAs were adjusting to HITECH's changes to the accounting of disclosures requirement, HHS published a proposed rule per an NPRM on May 31, 2011 (HIPAA Privacy Rule Accounting of Disclosures Under the Health Information Technology for Economic and Clinical Health Act) that proposed to significantly alter the accounting of disclosures requirement from both the original HIPAA implementation (2003) and HITECH (2009).

Per the NPRM, the accounting of disclosures right would be divided into two parts by creating a new "access report" applicable to EHRs and electronic PHI in a designated record set (AHIMA 2011). An individual, then, would be able to access two distinct reports: the accounting of disclosures report (which applies to paper and electronic PHI) and the access report (which applies to electronic PHI).

The **access report** would enable individuals to find out who has accessed their electronic PHI, including persons who accessed it as part of their routine work (AHIMA 2011). (Note that this differs from an accounting of disclosures, which only pertains to PHI that has been disclosed, not that which has been accessed through a use.) Under this proposed rule, covered entities would be encouraged to use access logs and audit trails (including systems maintained by its BAs) to generate user-friendly access reports. Key characteristics of the access report are outlined in figure 6.5.

Figure 6.6 provides a full set of provision comparisons among the accounting of disclosures as it originally existed per HIPAA; the changes to the accounting of disclosures as set forth by HITECH; and the changes created by the proposed access report in the May 31, 2011 NPRM. It provides a longitudinal description of the revisions set forth by HITECH and how the NPRM makes significant changes, particularly with the exclusion of uses and TPO from the accounting of disclosures because of the addition of the proposed access report.

FIGURE 6.5.	Characteristics of an access report

Applies to EHRs and electronic PHI
Includes both uses and disclosures
Includes TPO
Includes electronic PHI accessed during the prior three years
Must be generated within 30 days, with one 30-day extension
Includes, for each episode of access:

- Date and time of access
- What electronic PHI was accessed
- Who accessed the electronic PHI
- Description of access (for example, view, print, edit) if available

Source: AHIMA 2011

FIGURE 6.6.	Comparison of accounting of disclosures under HIPAA, HITECH, and May 31, 2011 NPRM (with access report)

HIPAA (CFR 164.528)	ARRA/HITECH (February 2009)	May 31, 2011 NPRM
No difference between paper and electronic (with either medium, TPO does *not* have to be accounted for)	TPO must be accounted for by covered entities with EHRs; requirement dates vary based on when the EHR is implemented (for EHRs acquired before 1/1/09, effective date is 1/1/14; for EHRs acquired after 1/1/09, effective date was 1/1/11)	Uses and TPO excluded from accounting of disclosures (for both paper and electronic) (Note: This apparent reversal from HITECH's position is due to the fact that the access report would include this information)

FIGURE 6.6. (Continued)		
HIPAA (CFR 164.528)	**ARRA/HITECH (February 2009)**	**May 31, 2011 NPRM**
Must account for previous *six* years' disclosures	Must account for previous *three* years' disclosures	No change from HITECH
List of exceptions to the accounting requirement is provided	No change from HIPAA	List of what is to be *included* in an accounting is to be provided
All PHI	No change from HIPAA	PHI in DRS only
No access report	No change from HIPAA	"Access report" (separate from disclosure report) added (applicable to EHRs) to allow individuals to see every person who has viewed the individual's DRS in the previous three years; some TPO disclosure information moved from disclosure report to access report
60 days to respond to accounting request, with one 30-day extension	No change from HIPAA	30 days to respond to accounting request, with one 30-day extension
Must account for all disclosures not authorized by patient (with certain exceptions)	No change from HIPAA	Exclusions for: (a) abuse, neglect, domestic violence; (b) health oversight; (c) research; (d) decedents; (e) protective services of president; (f) required by law (except courts or law enforcement)
Information contained in disclosure report	No changes from HIPAA	Specificity of information relaxed

Minimum Necessary (Section 13405)

Minimum necessary has been a requirement since HIPAA first went into effect. However, the interpretation of its definition, the amount needed "to accomplish the intended purpose" (45 CFR 164.502(b)), has been somewhat unclear depending on who is making the determination about what should be used or disclosed. HITECH has sought to clarify the definition of "minimum necessary" through guidance from the Secretary of HHS.

Clarification is still pending. Until a final determination is made, covered entities are instructed to use the limited data set (that is, PHI with certain specified direct identifiers removed, as described in chapter 2) as a guideline for using or disclosing only the minimum necessary information. In the meantime, if the limited data set is inadequate, covered entities are instructed to revert back to the "amount needed to accomplish the intended purpose" definition (AHIMA 2009). The January 2013 final rule is clear that the minimum necessary standard now applies to BAs (AHIMA 2013). Further guidance for minimum necessary is expected to be issued on the OCR website.

PHR Vendors (Section 13407)

As described in the BA section, PHR vendors may be considered BAs. They can also be noncovered entities and non-BAs. This could occur if they do not meet the definition of a covered entity and are not using or disclosing PHI on behalf of a covered entity, but are nonetheless providing a service where individuals create and store their PHRs. Noncovered entities and non-BAs (including PHR vendors, third-party service providers of PHR vendors, and other non-HIPAA covered entities or BAs affiliated with PHR vendors) must comply with companion breach notification regulations issued by the Federal Trade Commission (FTC) on August 25, 2009. The FTC regulations are similar to the HHS regulations in that, under both sets, entities must identify breaches and make appropriate notifications. In particular, entities subject to FTC regulations must notify the FTC and the individual(s) affected by the breach. Third-party PHR service providers shall notify the PHR vendor or entity of the breach. Other notification requirements, such as the content and nature of breach notices, are parallel to the HHS requirements (AHIMA 2009).

FIGURE 6.7.	Exceptions to the HITECH marketing definition

- Communications for treatment, including case management and care coordination, or to recommend alternatives (if no compensation)
- To provide refill reminders or communicate about a currently prescribed drug (compensation permitted, but is an exception only if compensation is reasonably related to the covered entity's cost)
- Healthcare operation activities (if no compensation):
  - that describe a health-related product or service included in a plan of benefits, or add value (but are not part of) a plan of benefits, or
  - that are case management and care coordination about treatment alternatives (and which do not fall within the treatment definition)

Source: AHIMA 2010 and AHIMA 2013

Marketing (Section 13406)

As a general rule, HIPAA identifies **marketing** as a communication by a covered entity or BA about a product or service that encourages recipients to purchase or use it (45 CFR 164.501). Activities that are considered marketing under HIPAA have generally required an authorization for use and disclosure. Conversely, healthcare operations have not required an authorization. Since HIPAA originally went into effect, covered entities and BAs have defined many activities as healthcare operations, either in good faith or in order to avoid the marketing authorization requirements.

HITECH strengthens limits on the use and disclosures of PHI by expanding activities defined as marketing and limits the definition of healthcare operations. The goal is to curtail current marketing practices and increase the numbers and types of activities for which authorization is required for use and disclosure to occur. Per HITECH, the situations listed in figure 6.7 are specifically listed as exceptions to marketing (and authorization is therefore not required). HITECH requires that any financial remuneration (compensation) received in exchange for marketing must be clearly disclosed in authorizations that are obtained, of course, prior to the communications. Financial remuneration includes direct and indirect payment (that is, on behalf of a third party), but it does not include non-financial in-kind benefits (AHIMA 2013).

Fundraising (Section 13406)

HITECH has imposed additional requirements on covered entities with respect to **fundraising**, limiting the use and disclosure of PHI and giving individuals greater rights in the process. Per HITECH, fundraising communications use or disclose PHI that are considered healthcare operations and that are sent to individuals must "clearly and conspicuously" provide a way to opt out of any future fundraising communications (AHIMA 2009). "Clearly and conspicuously" is not defined in HITECH. If fundraising solicitations do not stem from PHI (for example, a public directory is used to target individuals living in a particular area), HITECH's fundraising provisions do not apply (AHIMA 2013). Although HIPAA required that efforts be made to prevent further fundraising notifications when the individual did not want to receive them, HITECH strengthens an individual's ability to opt out of receiving fundraising solicitations by stating that the opt-out is to be treated as a revocation of authorization and no further fundraising communications may be made (although the covered entity can decide if the

FIGURE 6.8.	Exceptions to the HITECH sale of information authorization requirements

- For public health activities
- For research activities (and the price reflects the cost of preparation and data transmittal)
- For treatment and payment
- Related to sale, transfer, merger, or consolidation of all or part of a covered entity related to due diligence
- To provide an individual with a copy of his or her PHI
- By a covered entity to a BA pursuant to a BAA
- If deemed necessary and appropriate by the Secretary of HHS, or as required by law
- For other permitted purposes with reasonable, cost-based remuneration, or where the fee is expressly permitted by law

Source: ARRA 2009, 45 CFR 164.501(2006), and AHIMA 2013

prohibition applies to this campaign only, or permanently). Treatment or payment may not be conditioned on an individual's decision about receiving fundraising communications. Individuals must be notified, in the Notice of Privacy Practices, that they may receive fundraising communications. However, opt-out opportunities prior to the first solicitation are not required (AHIMA 2009 and AHIMA 2013).

Sale of Information (Section 13405)

HIPAA did not directly prohibit the **sale of information**. HITECH has changed this by now imposing new restrictions on the sale of information. HITECH states that a covered entity or BA may not sell (that is, receive compensation for) any PHI without a valid authorization from the individual. There are exceptions. These are listed in figure 6.8. If an authorization is required (and signed by the individual), it must state whether the individual permits or prohibits the entity receiving the PHI to further exchange it for compensation. In contrast with the definition of remuneration per the HIPAA marketing provisions, remuneration does include non-financial (in-kind) benefits. Fees generated for a profit are not allowed (AHIMA 2013).

Increased Enforcement and Penalties (Sections 13409, 13410, 13411)

A number of changes to enforcement and penalty provisions for HIPAA violations have been brought about by HITECH. Although corrective action continues to serve a covered entity or BA well, overall there is a notable movement away from a collaborative approach to a more punitive stance. HITECH, through both the February 2009 HITECH legislation and the October 2009 interim final rule on enforcement, revised the 2006 **Enforcement Rule**, which had created standardized procedures and substantive requirements for investigating complaints and imposing civil monetary penalties for HIPAA violations, including privacy and security violations (Brodnik et al. 2012). The January 2013 final rule adopted the October 2009 interim final rule (AHIMA 2013).

This section will discuss HITECH changes including the involvement of state Attorneys General, audits, individual prosecution, tiered penalties, and individual compensation.

Attorneys General (Section 13410)

HITECH grants state attorneys general the ability, per their *parens patriae* power, or authority to act on their citizens' behalf, to bring civil actions in federal district court on behalf of individuals believed to have been negatively affected by a HIPAA violation. Previously, only the **Office of Civil Rights (OCR)** for HHS, which enforces HIPAA, held this right (and individuals still cannot bring lawsuits under HIPAA). The OCR encourages collaboration with state attorneys general and, to promote this, it provided specialized HIPAA training to attorneys general in the spring and summer of 2011. As of this publication, few actions had been brought but an increase in lawsuits may be seen. Cases that have been brought are outlined as follows:

- In January 2010, the attorney general of Connecticut brought a federal (HIPAA) action against health plan HealthNet following the loss of a portable computer disk containing unencrypted information (Center for Public Integrity 2011). The case was settled for $250,000.

- In January 2011, the attorney general of Vermont brought an action against health plan HealthNet. This action focused on the health plan's failure to promptly notify of a breach of PHI of 1.5 million people, including 525 Vermont residents. The case settled for $55,000 (Center for Public Integrity 2011). It was brought under both federal law (HIPAA) and Vermont state law.

- In January 2012, the Minnesota attorney general brought an action against Accretive Health, a BA that managed collections for several Minnesota hospitals. This action stemmed from the theft of a laptop from a car in July 2011. The laptop contained unencrypted information about 23,500 individuals. The case settled for $2.5 million and Accretive agreed not to conduct business in Minnesota for two years. The case was brought under both federal law (HIPAA) and state law. Although the action was based on the theft of PHI, the case was also impacted by Accretive's allegedly aggressive collections tactics (Chicago Tribune 2012). This case was the first enforcement action brought directly against a BA for violating its HITECH obligations.

Audits (Section 13411)

Prior to HITECH, detection of HIPAA violations was solely complaint driven. As such, enforcement efforts were often criticized as "lacking teeth." HITECH provided for the Secretary of HHS to authorize periodic audits to determine covered entity and BA compliance with HIPAA (AHIMA 2009). In 2011, OCR contracted with KPMG, a public accounting firm, to conduct 150 audits by the end of 2012. As of publication, the first 20 audits have been completed and included health plans, healthcare clearinghouses, and numerous types of providers including hospitals, physician offices, and one each of the following: laboratory, dental office, nursing home, and pharmacy. The initial plan to conduct 150 audits was modified, with only 95 more audits to be completed by the end of 2012. It was announced that BAs will be included in future audits.

Audits consist of a notification or preparation phase, with 10 days to produce required documentation and a minimum of 30 days to prepare for the on-site visit. The visit itself is anywhere from three to ten days and includes interviews with key personnel and observations of processes and operations to determine compliance. A draft report is shared with the covered entity at the end of the survey, and a final report is submitted to OCR incorporating corrective action steps needed by the covered entity.

Individual Prosecution (Section 13409)

Section 13409 of HITECH amends Section 1177(a) of the Social Security Act, which addresses criminal penalties associated with the wrongful disclosure of individually identifiable information. HITECH clarifies that a person, including an employee or other individual, may be criminally prosecuted for HIPAA privacy and security violations (AHIMA 2009). This changes the previous HIPAA position that covered entities, but not their employees, could be prosecuted.

Tiered Penalties (Section 13410)

HITECH has increased civil monetary penalties based on levels of intent and neglect. These are **tiered penalties**. Maximum penalties are based on repeated violations within a year's time. The tiers are:

- Unknowing or did not know (and would not have known that a violation was committed, even with reasonable diligence): $100–$50,000 per violation (maximum $1,500,000 in a calendar year for identical violations)

- Reasonable cause (an act or omission in which a covered entity or BA knew, or with reasonable diligence would have known, of a violation, but it cannot be identified as willful neglect): $1,000–$50,000 per violation (maximum $1,500,000 in a calendar year for identical violations)

- Willful neglect:
  - ◆ $10,000–$50,000 per violation (maximum $1,500,000 in a calendar year for identical violations) if corrected
  - ◆ $50,000 per violation (maximum $1,500,000 in a calendar year for identical violations) if uncorrected (AHIMA 2009)

The nature and extent of both the violation and the harm, including number of individuals involved, time period in which the violations occurred, reputational harm, and prior indicators of noncompliance are considered to determine the amount assessed within each range. The OCR has discretion to pursue corrective action without assessing penalties for unknowing violations (and where reasonable diligence would not have revealed the violation). Where willful neglect is found, civil penalties are required (AHIMA 2013). Penalty monies collected will support further enforcement efforts (AHIMA 2009 and AHIMA 2013).

Individual Compensation (Section 13410)

HITECH provided that a method for compensating individuals harmed by a HIPAA violation would be recommended to the Secretary of HHS. The method introduced in HITECH would compensate the individual with a percentage of the civil monetary penalty or monetary settlement collected. A proposed rule regarding such compensation has not yet been published.

Provisions First Introduced in NPRMs

The following provisions were not present in HITECH originally, but were first introduced in proposed rules that were published in subsequent NPRMs. The final rule for the July 2010 proposed rule was sent to OMB in March 2012. OMB is given 90 to 120 days to review final rules, but a publication of the final rule in the Federal Register was delayed until January 25, 2013. The May 2011 proposed rule for Accounting of Disclosures is still pending. No definite date has been announced for publication of the final rule subsequent to the May 2011 proposed rule. The proposed rules (and dates of NPRMs) in which each of the following provisions were included are listed in the following sections.

PHI of Decedents (July 14, 2010 NPRM)

Although not introduced under the original HITECH legislation, the July 2010 proposed rule included a new provision regarding the PHI of decedents. Affirmed by the January 2013 final rule individually identifiable health information of persons deceased for more than 50 years is no longer PHI and no longer is protected by the Privacy Rule. The PHI does not have to be retained 50 years if organizational policy provides for its destruction at an earlier time. Further, this provision does not override more protective state laws (AHIMA 2013). The proposed rule also enabled access to PHI of a deceased individual family members or others who were involved in the decedent's care or payment prior to the decedent's death, unless the disclosure would be inconsistent with known previously stated wishes of the decedent (AHIMA 2010). This was also affirmed by the January 2013 final rule, although such disclosure is permissive and not mandatory (AHIMA 2013).

Research Authorization Requirements (July 14, 2010 NPRM)

The July 2010 rule proposed, and the January 2013 final rule confirmed, changes to research authorization requirements so that HIPAA does not impede progress in research studies. A conditioned authorization (that is, one that conditions the provision of research-related treatment on the provision of an authorization) and an unconditioned authorization can be combined for research as long as the authorization clearly differentiates the two and clearly allows the individual to opt in to unconditioned research activities. This provision does not apply, however, to research involving use or disclosure of psychotherapy notes. Psychotherapy note authorizations cannot be combined with other authorizations. The final rule also permits authorizations for future research use or disclosure in order to limit the burden of additional authorizations for secondary research that may not be able to be anticipated at the time the authorization was signed (AHIMA 2010 and AHIMA 2013).

Student Immunization Records (July 14, 2010 NPRM)

The January 2013 final rule makes it easier for schools to receive student immunization records where state or other law requires it prior to a student being admitted. Prior to the January 2010 proposed rule, written authorization was required for this PHI to be disclosed. Now a covered entity's disclosure of immunization records to schools is considered a public health disclosure, which does not require written authorization from either the student's parent or guardian (or student, if the student is an adult or otherwise able to authorize). Oral agreement from the parent, guardian, or student is still required. The oral agreement must be documented, demonstrating that the records were received per this provision; however, no signature is required (AHIMA 2013).

The goal is to facilitate compliance with state laws that require proof of immunization for children enrolling in school.

Notice of Privacy Practices (July 14, 2010 NPRM and May 31, 2011 NPRM)

Changes will have to be made to **notices of privacy practices** in order to reflect new requirements. Specifically, notices will have to be updated to

- Address changes to individual rights to include the right to be notified of a breach of unsecured PHI if they are affected
- State that uses and disclosures not described in the notice will require an authorization
- State (if applicable to the organization) that most uses and disclosures of psychotherapy notes will require an authorization
- Reflect changes to marketing, fundraising, and sale of information requirements
- State that restriction requests must be honored for items or services paid by the individual in full out of pocket (AHIMA 2010, 2011)

Providers do not have to print and distribute the revised NPP to all individuals who seek treatment. However, it must be posted prominently and copies must be available for individuals to take, without having to ask for them. As has always been the case, the NPP must continue to be given to new patients.

CHECK YOUR UNDERSTANDING 6.2

Instructions: Indicate whether the following statements are true or false (T or F).

1. HITECH gives state attorneys general the power to bring civil actions in federal district court on behalf of residents negatively affected by a HIPAA violation.

2. Per HITECH, covered entities never have to agree to individuals' requests to restrict uses and disclosures of PHI for carrying out TPO.

3. The penalty amount for a violation of HIPAA due to willful neglect is the same whether the violation was corrected or not.

4. According to the January 2013 final rulemaking, PHI of a decedent loses its PHI status 50 years after the individual's death.

5. The access report proposed by the May 31, 2011 Notice of Proposed Rulemaking would include both uses and disclosures of PHI.

REAL-WORLD CASE

In February 2011, the Office of Civil Rights (OCR) for HHS issued its first civil monetary penalty to a covered entity for HIPAA Privacy Rule violations. Prior to this, offenders had agreed to change their business practices or had entered into settlement agreements with

OCR. This case also represented application of the tiered penalties authorized by section 13410 of HITECH.

Cignet Health was a healthcare provider that operated two clinics in Maryland. The HIPAA rights of 41 patients were violated when Cignet repeatedly denied the patients access to their health records. After the patients submitted complaints to OCR, Cignet refused to comply with OCR's investigation including failure to respond to a subpoena from OCR. Cignet's actions were deemed to be willful neglect as defined under HITECH. Cignet's $4.3 million penalty was due to willful neglect: $1.3 million for failure to grant patients access to their records, and $3 million for failure to cooperate with the government's investigation.

OCR used this case to emphasize that covered entities and business associates have a responsibility to comply with HIPAA's requirements. It further cautioned against knowingly disregarding obligations under HIPAA (HHS 2011).

SUMMARY

HITECH was passed as part of the American Recovery and Reinvestment Act in February 2009. Although HITECH provided significant funding to promote health information technology, it also made significant changes to HIPAA. This chapter discussed HITECH's original changes to HIPAA (February 2009), interim final rules relative to breach notification and enforcement, published in August 2009 and October 2009, respectively, and proposed rules in July 2010 and May 2011 that made even further significant changes. A final rule published January 25, 2013 finalized changes in the two interim final rules and the 2010 proposed rule, with an effective date of March 26, 2013. Other proposed HITECH changes, particularly relating to the May 2011 proposed rule, are still pending.

HITECH requires significant operational changes to maintain compliance. However, its greatest impact is likely in the form of its scope and potential penalties. Business associates are now obligated to comply with HIPAA simply by meeting the definition of a business associate. No longer is a contract (that is, a business associate agreement) required to legally bind a business associate to HIPAA's requirements. Further, covered entities and business associates alike face much greater penalties for noncompliance. This punitive approach is likely a direct response to criticisms about HIPAA's "lack of teeth." HITECH has also expanded individuals' rights through requirements related to breach notification, access, restriction requests, and use of PHI for marketing and fundraising. These are but a few of the changes brought about by HITECH. With an increase in responsibilities and greater risks associated with failure to comply, covered entities and business associates are challenged to stay abreast of HITECH's requirements.

REFERENCES

American Health Information Management Association. 2013. Analysis of Modifications to the HIPAA Privacy, Security, Enforcement, and Breach Notification Rules Under the Health Information Technology for Economic and Clinical Health Act and the Genetic Information Nondiscrimination Act; Other Modifications to the HIPAA Rules. http://library.ahima.org/xpedio/groups/public/documents/ahima/bok1_050067.pdf.

American Health Information Management Association. 2012. *Pocket Glossary for Health Information Management and Technology*, 3rd ed. Chicago: AHIMA.

American Health Information Management Association. 2011. Analysis of the Proposed Rule, May 31, 2011, HIPAA Privacy Rule Accounting of Disclosures under the Health Information Technology for Economic and Clinical Health Act (HITECH). http://www.ahima.org/downloads/pdfs/advocacy/Analysis_of_the_NPRM_HITECH_AoD(fin).pdf.

American Health Information Management Association. 2010. Overview of the Proposed Rule: Modifications to the HIPAA Privacy, Security, and Enforcement Rules under the Health Information Technology for Economic and Clinical Health Act. http://www.ahima.org/downloads/pdfs/advocacy/Analysis%20of%20Privacy%20Rule%20Fule%20Content%20fin%20.pdf.

American Health Information Management Association. 2009. Analysis of Healthcare Confidentiality, Privacy, and Security Provisions of the American Recovery and Reinvestment Act of 2009, Public Law 111-5. http://www.ahima.org/downloads/pdfs/advocacy/AnalysisofARRAPrivacy-fin-3-2009a.pdf.

American Recovery and Reinvestment Act of 2009. Title XIII: Health Information Technology, Subtitle D: Privacy, Part 1: Improved Privacy Provisions and Security Provisions, Sections 13401–13411.

Brodnik, M., L. Rinehart-Thompson, and R. Reynolds. 2012. *Fundamentals of Law for Health Informatics and Information Management*. Chicago: AHIMA.

Center for Public Integrity. 2011. State attorneys general not leaping to embrace HIPAA enforcement. http://www.iwatchnews.org/2011/09/20/6666/state-attorneys-general-not-leaping-embrace-hipaa-enforcement.

Chicago Tribune. 2012 (July 30). Accretive settles Minnesota charges for $2.5M. http://articles.chicagotribune.com/2012-07-30/business/chi-accretive-settles-minnesota-charges-for-25m-20120730_1_accretive-health-mary-tolan-fairview-hospitals.

Copeland, Curtis W. 2011. The Federal Rulemaking Process: An Overview. CRS Report for Congress. Congressional Research Service. http://www.thecre.com/pdf/20120422_RL32240.pdf.

Department of Health and Human Services. 2012. Health Information Privacy. Breaches Affecting 500 or More Individuals. http://www.hhs.gov/ocr/privacy/hipaa/administrative/breachnotificationrule/breachtool.html.

Department of Health and Human Services. 2011. HHS imposes a $4.3 million civil monetary penalty for violations of the HIPAA Privacy Rule. http://www.hhs.gov/news/press/2011pres/02/20110222a.html.

Department of Health and Human Services. 2009. Breach Notification for Unsecured Protected Health Information; Interim Final Rule. 45 CFR Parts 160 and 164. *Federal Register* 74(162): 42740–42770.

45 CFR 164.501: Privacy of individually identifiable health information. Definitions. 2006.

45 CFR 164.502(b): Standard: minimum necessary. 2006.

5 USC §551 et seq.: Administrative Procedure Act. 1946.

Appendix A

PRIVACY OFFICER

Sample Position Description

General Purpose: The privacy officer oversees all activities related to the development, implementation, maintenance of, and adherence to the organization's privacy program in compliance with federal and state laws and industry standards. Activities include developing policies and procedures, as well as workforce educational activities that address access, use, and disclosure of patient health information.

Reports to: Chief Information Officer or Vice President of Corporate Compliance

Responsibilities

Oversight of the Privacy Program

- Develop, implement, and maintain the organization's protected health information privacy and security policies, procedures and guidelines in compliance with federal and state laws, as well as accreditation standards, and in coordination with organization leadership, the Privacy compliance oversight structure, and legal counsel

- Set the direction and provide the vision for the privacy compliance program. Plans, implements, and directs ongoing privacy and data security risk activities

- Report on the status of the privacy and data security program

- Measure effectiveness, performance and quality of the program to the board, system leadership and Privacy compliance oversight structure as well as provide input, recommendations, and guidance on privacy and security issues

- Collaborate and coordinate with the Security Officer for ongoing compliance auditing and monitoring programs involving workforce members, business associates, trading partners, and such to ensure that organizational privacy and security policies and procedures are up-to-date and maintained addressing concerns, requirements, and responsibilities

Compliance

- Establishes, resolves, and administers a process for the receipt, documentation, receiving, tracking, and investigation of compliance violations against the organization's privacy and data security practices as well as provide recommendations and execute actions for said violations.

- Investigates and monitors all complaints to ensure the consistent application of sanctions for failure to comply with privacy practices

- Reviews all organizational information security and privacy plans to ensure alignment between security and privacy practices

- Collaborates with leadership, key departments, and committees or structures to ensure the implementation, maintenance, enforcement, and update of appropriate documentation (for example, NPP, authorization forms, investigation forms, and such) as needed in compliance with federal laws, state laws, and relevant accreditation standards

- Performs or directs risk assessments (that is, protected information privacy and security audits, policies and procedures, trend analyses, audits, projects, and violation investigations) to ensure organizational compliance

- Ensures organizational compliance with legal, ethical, regulatory, accreditation, licensing, certification requirements, and other administrative requirements regarding privacy and data security, and implementation of supporting administrative, physical, and technical safeguards

- Cooperates with the Office for Civil Rights and other investigative agencies in coordination with organization officers in responding to external compliance reviews or investigations

Daily Operations
- Facilitates privacy and security training through awareness activities providing education on organizational policies, procedures, and practices

- Serves on various committees and projects in a leadership role for the planning, design, and evaluation of privacy, and data security; coordinates development of strategic teams, work groups, and resources

- Delegates responsibility and authority to individuals to act as privacy and data security coordinators as needed

- Directs and manages the daily operations of privacy and collaborates with the Security Officer to ensure data security compliance

- Develops job descriptions, manages budgets and performs financial processes, strategic planning, and staff management functions

- Provide leadership, strategic direction, and affirms that the workforce of the organization adheres to regulatory mandates regarding privacy and confidentiality

Exchange of Information
- Directs the development and management of the organization's authorization forms and release of information policies, procedures, and practices for disclosure of PHI; responds to requests to exercise individual's privacy rights (that is, inspection, amendment, account of disclosures, and restriction of access to PHI).

- Ensures the efficiency and efficacy of the organization's processes with respect to the electronic exchange of data and patient information in compliance with state and federal laws.

- Designs, implements, and manages role-based access control; oversees audits of access to PHI; recommends appropriate action necessary as a result of audit activities

Privacy Expertise
- Serves as primary liaison to the community on federal and state regulations such as Privacy, IRB, and clinical and administrative systems. Serve as secondary liaison (under security officer) on any Data Security topics (as needed).

- Serve as an internal resource or consultant to the organization on privacy compliance related activities and serves as backup to the Security Officer when needed on security compliance related activities.
- Work with organization leadership, legal counsel, the Security Officer, and other related parties to represent the organization's information privacy and security interests with external parties who undertake to adopt or amend privacy legislation, regulations, or standards
- Maintain current knowledge of applicable federal and state health information privacy and security laws and accreditation standards
- Monitors advancements in information privacy technology to ensure organizational adaptation and compliance
- Provides community support for privacy and security initiatives that impact the organization and its stakeholders

Other Skills

- Proficient in Microsoft Office: PC-based spreadsheet programs (for example, Power Point, Excel, Word)
- Knowledge of and the ability to apply the principles of HIM, project management, and change management; knowledge of health care industry
- Demonstrates organization, facilitation, communication, and presentation skills
- Experience in information systems and data risk management
- Internal investigative experience preferred
- High degree of personal and professional integrity

Requirements

- Bachelor's degree in Health Information Management, Healthcare Administration, or related field required. Master's degree preferred.
- CHPS, RHIA, or RHIT credential preferred.
- At least five years in healthcare operations, clinical care, health information management, research, or a related field.

Notes

1. The title for this position will vary from organization to organization, and may not be the primary title of the individual serving in the position. "Chief" would most likely refer to very large integrated delivery systems. The term "privacy officer" is specifically mentioned in the HIPAA/HITECH Privacy Regulation.
2. The reporting structure for this position will vary depending on the institution and its size. Since many of the functions are already inherent in the Health Information or Medical Records Department or function, many organizations may elect to keep this function in that department.

Appendix B

HEALTHCARE INFORMATION SECURITY OFFICER

Sample Job Description

General Purpose: The security officer is responsible for the design, oversight, and ongoing management of the information security program, including policies, procedures, technical systems, and workforce training in order to maintain the confidentiality, integrity, and availability of data within all healthcare organization information systems. The security officer role addresses electronic systems architecture and functionality as it affects safeguards of protected health information (PHI) and business information assets.

Reports to: Varies (recommend reporting to the C-Level)

General Responsibilities

Responsibilities include management of system technology to support information privacy and security requirements; maintenance of confidentiality, integrity, and availability of data as the privacy and security programs integrate; development and maintenance of security policies and procedures including management of security risk assessments, the program budget, security complaints and incident activity, and enforcement; workforce security training and awareness; application of industry standards and best practices; external compliance assurances and security survey activity; and business continuity planning. The security official serves as the security voice on the Privacy and Security Committee or Council for decision-making around information security decisions for internal and health information exchange business decisions.

Daily Operations

- Responsible for implementing, managing and enforcing information security derivatives within regulatory mandates to protect PHI including HIPAA and The American Recovery and Reinvestment Act provisions
- Ensure the ongoing integration of information security with business strategies and privacy requirements
- Work closely with the organization's privacy officer for ongoing optimal application of technology functionality to protect PHI, including the identity management program
- Lead information security awareness and training initiatives to educate workforce about policies, procedures and information risks
- Conduct risk analyses to assess the probability of risks occurring and the impact on the organization
- Create an information security risk mitigation plan based on sound risk analysis

- Perform ongoing security audits to assess effectiveness or policies or procedures and systems security safeguards
- Work with contractual and other activities with vendors, outside consultants, business associates, and other third parties to improve information security practices
- Lead the security incident response team in prevention, investigation, mitigation, and reporting activities; ensure appropriate enforcement sanctions for information security breaches
- Responsible for budget-related activities for the security program

Performance Improvement

- Manage complaint and incident preventative and investigative programs related to security policies
- Carry out periodic security risk assessments in conjunction with privacy requirements
- Manage the security audit program; coordinate action plans for applicable departments when necessary to make improvements
- Responsible for documenting and maintaining all risk analysis and remediation actions taken by the organization to reduce information security risks
- Manage retention of performance improvement activity documentation for security functions and compliance responsibilities
- Recommend system enhancements via capital and operational budget planning to keep pace with privacy and security technology advances
- Coordinate security survey regulatory activities and participates in accreditation surveys with external survey bodies

Knowledge and Skills

- Maintain current knowledge of
    - Federal and state privacy and security laws and regulations
    - Industry best practices (that is, NIST, ISO)
- Manage the security of health information across a widely dispersed workforce with a variety of information mediums
- Capability to serve as a security resource to all levels including executive management, department employees, business associates, and external bodies such as state agencies
- Demonstrate leadership qualities toward health reform progress, interoperability preparedness, and health information exchange progression
- Provide project management oversight and operational responsibility for administrative coordination and implementation of the organization's security program
- Demonstrate competence in the areas of the critical thinking and problem solving, interpersonal relationships, and technical skills

Qualifications

- Bachelor's in Information Systems, Computer Science, Health Information Management, or related field
- Five years experience in healthcare-related fields, demonstrated expertise in healthcare operations, health information knowledge, change management, and project management
- Security certification preferred: Certified Information System Security Professional (CISSP), Certified Information Systems Manager (CISM), Certified in Healthcare Privacy and Security (CHPS)
- Previous work experience preferred with federal and state privacy and security laws, regulations, and accreditation standards for maintaining information security and confidentiality
- Leadership qualities with knowledge of technical infrastructure security components and integrated, computerized rules-based systems

Appendix C

HIPAA PRIVACY AND SECURITY CASE STUDIES

Many of the case studies in this appendix are adapted from Thomason, Mary. 2008. *HIPAA by Example*. Chicago: AHIMA. They are noted as such.

Should the *Town Square Times* Be Concerned about the HIPAA Privacy Rule?

The *Town Square Times*, a local newspaper, issued a statement that it could no longer publish birth information unless it was accompanied by a signed authorization from the mother because birth information is protected health information (PHI) per HIPAA. Up to this point, birth information had typically been submitted directly to the newspaper by proud grandparents.

One of the first questions is whether the situation involves a covered entity. Covered entities include healthcare providers, health plans, and healthcare clearinghouses. A newspaper is none of the three. The newspaper is correct that birth information is (PHI) per HIPAA. Also, as a matter of policy, the *Town Square Times* may decide to protect the privacy of its local parents and newborns who might not otherwise appreciate submissions by family members. However, the newspaper is not bound by HIPAA and need not worry that it is committing a HIPAA violation. If birth information is also submitted to the newspaper by hospitals where the births occurred, the hospitals would need to be certain they had obtained the appropriate authorizations for disclosure of birth information because they are covered entities. Again, however, this need not be the newspaper's concern.

Is a Volunteer Emergency Medical Services Unit a Covered Entity?

Mary is a member of a volunteer emergency medical services (EMS) unit in the fire department of a small, rural town. The town does not have much money and has never invested in resources to determine whether it should comply with HIPAA. In addition, it has only one computer terminal that is used for the sole purpose of logging and storing emergency run data. Recently, Mary mentioned that perhaps they should see if HIPAA applies to them, particularly because of recent media reports of "big penalties" for noncompliance. The senior member of the EMS unit said HIPAA does not apply to them because they are just a small volunteer organization, unlike hospitals and physician offices.

The senior member could be right, but his reasoning is incorrect. An EMS unit is a healthcare provider. However, not all healthcare providers are covered entities. For HIPAA to apply, healthcare providers must conduct certain electronic transactions (such as transmission of health claims). The EMS unit must evaluate whether or not it conducts any of these electronic transactions. It appears that it does not. The computer is used only to log and store information (no electronic transmissions are mentioned). Of further note, as a volunteer department it may be supported solely by taxpayer dollars and might not bill for its services at all.

Does the HIPAA Privacy Rule Apply to Health Fairs?

The HIPAA Privacy Rule can apply where a covered entity creates, maintains, transmits, or receives individually identifiable health information. Covered entities such as hospitals and clinics that participate in health fairs may not collect information at all or they may collect individually identifiable information unrelated to a person's health information (for example, to conduct a raffle). In either case, no PHI is involved so the HIPAA Privacy Rule would not apply. However, if health information is collected or somehow is linked to individuals' PHI in the covered entity's possession (with, perhaps, the goal of marketing products and services to the individuals), the HIPAA Privacy Rule does apply. Another common health fair activity of healthcare providers is to conduct screening tests for visitors. If results are merely given to the visitor without being recorded, HIPAA does not apply. On the other hand, if the covered entity records and keeps individually identifiable records that presumably would be related to treatment purposes, HIPAA does apply. Once the Privacy Rule applies, a covered entity must give an individual a Notice of Privacy Practices if this is the first encounter with the covered entity (Thomason 2008).

Does the HIPAA Privacy Rule Apply to Flu Shot Clinics?

The HIPAA Privacy Rule can apply where a covered entity creates, maintains, or receives or transmits individually identifiable health information. If the organization providing the flu shots is not a covered entity, HIPAA does not apply. For example, an employer may provide a flu shot clinic as a service to its employees. However, the employer may not be a covered entity. Another common example is a public health department, which often provides flu shot clinics. However, a public health department may or may not be a covered entity. Factors that influence its designation include whether it provides treatment or not (that is, whether it is a healthcare provider). If it provides treatment, if and how it is reimbursed for providing treatment must be considered and HIPAA may apply. If the public health department is not a covered entity because it does not qualify as a healthcare provider per HIPAA, it is not bound by HIPAA.

If an organization is determined to be a covered entity, whether or not HIPAA applies depends on the records it creates as part of its activity. If the covered entity generates or maintains identifiable results, for example, and notes them in a patient's clinic record, HIPAA applies and a Notice of Privacy Practices should be given to the individual receiving services for the first time.

A note about employers: Many employers are not covered entities; however, some are (such as hospitals and health plans). If a covered entity is conducting a flu shot clinic as a service to its employees as part of an employee health initiative, records created as a result of this employee health activity should be maintained in the employee health record. However, as long as the activity is performed by the employer as an employer (and not as a covered entity) and records are used for employment purposes only, HIPAA does not apply (Thomason 2008).

Are Court-Ordered Medical Evaluations Regulated under HIPAA?

Healthcare providers often perform court-ordered medical evaluations. If the healthcare provider is a covered entity, the evaluation is an activity that creates information about an individual's physical or mental health. However, if the covered entity does not use the findings in its evaluation to make decisions about the individual, one could argue that the information is not part of a designated record set. If, on the other hand, the covered entity uses the findings of the evaluation to care for the individual (this is common in behavioral health activities such as involuntary commitment hearings), the evaluation is now being used to make treatment decisions about the patient. In this case, the evaluation would be part of the designated record set and HIPAA applies. Because court-ordered evaluations are generated per the court's authority, the court may require the healthcare provider that performed the evaluation to disclose the results to the court or to other relevant entities. HIPAA permits such court-ordered disclosures, but applicable state laws and other federal laws must be considered as well. If those laws are more stringent (and thus provide greater privacy protections or greater patient rights), they must be followed. HIPAA only permits disclosures of this nature; it does not require them (Thomason 2008).

Are the Records of a Deceased Person Protected under HIPAA?

In general, the HIPAA Privacy Rule protects the health records of deceased individuals in the same way it protects health records of living individuals' records (although states may not protect records of the deceased under physician-patient privilege laws). Currently, HIPAA protects the information as long as the covered entity retains the records.

Note: Per the July 2010 proposed administrative rule, PHI of persons deceased for more than 50 years would lose its PHI status and no longer be protected by HIPAA (although covered entities would not be required to retain PHI for 50 years if their policies provide for earlier destruction). The proposed rule also stated that PHI of a deceased individual could be disclosed to a family member or others who were involved in the decedent's care or payment prior to the decedent's death, unless this would be inconsistent with wishes the decedent had previously made known. The January 2013 final rule affirmed this provision by excluding information about persons deceased more than 50 years from the PHI definition and permitting disclosure to family members as set forth in the proposed rule.

HIPAA allows funeral directors and coroners to receive PHI of decedents necessary to perform their duties, but applicable state laws and other federal laws must be considered as well. If those laws are more stringent (and thus provide greater privacy protections or greater patient rights), they must be followed. HIPAA only permits disclosures of this nature; it does not require them.

The right of access to a deceased individual's records is transferred to the individual's personal representative, which is usually the executor of the individual's estate. Additionally, HIPAA's research provisions allow research on decedents' records as long as a researcher certifies that the records required all belong to deceased patients (note that federal research regulations protect only human subjects and therefore do not extend to protect records of deceased individuals) (Thomason 2008).

Are Dates of Admission Protected Health Information?

Initially, a patient's dates of stay would not appear to fall within the HIPAA definition of PHI. However, HIPAA includes dates related to the individual as a data element that must be removed for deidentification. Prior to HIPAA, dates of admission were often disclosed to requesters without the individual's authorization. (These are still permitted, under the payment provision of treatment, payment and healthcare operations (TPO), to insurers who call to verify dates on submitted claims and to other requesters if the disclosure is for the purpose of treatment, payment, healthcare operations, or required by law. Disclosure of this information may also be made pursuant to individual authorization.)

Even if an individual is included in the facility directory, dates of admission cannot be provided. The purpose of the facility directory is to provide enough information (to those who ask about an individual by name) to locate the individual while he is in the facility, and to provide general information about the individual's condition.

Condition designations provided by the American Hospital Association are:

- Undetermined: Patient is awaiting physician and/or assessment.
- Good: Vital signs are stable and within normal limits. Patient is conscious and comfortable. Indicators are excellent.
- Fair: Vital signs are stable and within normal limits. Patient is conscious, but may be uncomfortable. Indicators are favorable.
- Serious: Vital signs may be unstable and not within normal limits. Patient is acutely ill. Indicators are questionable.
- Critical: Vital signs are unstable and not within normal limits. Patient may be unconscious. Indicators are unfavorable.

Admission dates are beyond the scope and purpose of the facility directory. One exception is a patient who calls to obtain his own admission dates. As long as the patient's identity can be verified, this information may be disclosed.

Applicable state laws and other federal laws must be considered as well. If those laws are more stringent (and thus provide greater privacy protections or greater patient rights), they must be followed. HIPAA only permits disclosures of this nature; it does not require them. In particular, there are specific rules for facilities bound by federal drug and alcohol treatment program regulations. The regulations do not allow programs to disclose that a patient has been treated in a program, without signed patient authorization. Facility directories are not advised for these types of programs (Thomason 2008).

Does the HIPAA Privacy Rule Require Us to Protect HIV or AIDS Patients' Records from Access within the Covered Entity?

HIPAA does not provide special protections based on diagnosis. All information is treated equally with the exception of the psychotherapy note, to which HIPAA applies special restrictions. HIPAA also provides individuals with the right to request restrictions on records (generally subject to covered entity agreement), but this right is not diagnosis-specific, either.

Diagnosis-specific protections (including HIV or AIDS) can be found in many state laws and generally require that very specific authorizations be signed by individuals before information can be disclosed. Many state laws also prohibit discrimination (for example, by health plans and employers) based on the receipt of diagnostic information such as HIV or AIDS (Thomason 2008).

Linda Is an At-Home, Independent Coding Professional Who Performs Coding Services for Two Small Physician Practices. One of the Practices Has Not Initiated a Business Associate Agreement (BAA) with Linda. Should She Be Concerned?

A business associate (BA) is person or organization who is not a member of a covered entity's workforce but performs certain functions on behalf of a covered entity that involve PHI. Linda meets HIPAA's definition of a BA. Prior to HITECH, Linda did not have a reason to be greatly concerned about the lack of a BAA. Because the physician's office failed to initiate this contract with her and therefore had not identified her as a BA, she was not bound to comply with HIPAA (although she could still be legally liable under applicable state laws for confidentiality breaches). Under HITECH, however, the nature of her work and her relationship with the physician's office (that is, using PHI on behalf of a covered entity) automatically qualifies her as a BA by law, even if no BAA has been signed. As such, she should be concerned because she is liable for HIPAA privacy and security violations, including breaches. Although she is not the covered entity, Linda should take steps to ensure that a BAA is completed and signed. The BAA should outline the agreement between the physician's office and Linda, including how PHI will be used and disclosed. With these details outlined in the BAA, Linda can be assured that she has the flexibility to do her job appropriately. Further, she will have been given explicit guidance about how to handle PHI.

May We Allow Our Facility Attorney to Review a Patient's Records in a Potential Litigation Case?

HIPAA permits a covered entity to disclose PHI for the healthcare operations of the covered entity. An individual's consent or authorization is not required. Conducting or arranging for legal services is specifically listed as a healthcare operation. The disclosure must be limited to the minimum necessary (note: of TPO, the minimum necessary requirement is lifted only for treatment purposes). As a member of the covered entity's workforce, the attorney is also obligated to only ask for the information needed. The attorney must also be reviewing the case for one of the covered entity's permitted uses. For example, the facility's attorney may review the PHI if a patient is thinking of suing because of alleged negligent treatment. However, the facility's attorney may not review PHI of a facility employee who is bringing an employment discrimination lawsuit against the facility.

Legal services can be provided by an attorney who is a member of the covered entity's workforce (as this scenario presented) or by an outside attorney serving as a BA (as long as the facility has a BAA with the attorney or his law firm).

Specific rules for facilities bound by federal drug and alcohol treatment program regulations must also be considered. They permit disclosure to an entity that has direct administrative control over a program, but the permitted disclosures appear to be limited to those necessary to provide the drug or alcohol treatment service. Because in-house legal review falls outside the treatment purview, patient authorization may be required. This may be challenging if the legal review is necessary because the patient is filing a lawsuit against the facility (Thomason 2008).

What Access Should Staff Members Have to the PHI of Patients Who Have Transferred to Other Units?

When patients are transferred from one hospital unit to another, staff members from the first unit often wish to continue accessing the transferred patients' PHI. Their intent is generally not malicious. They genuinely care about their patients and want to see that they are continuing to progress. Can the staff members from the first unit call the receiving unit or check the EHR to check on the patient or must access cease at the time of transfer?

While the staff members' caring attitudes are noble, they typically no longer have a need to access their former patients' PHI. Their access (and disclosure by the staff on the receiving units) are HIPAA violations. Additionally, inappropriate access to electronic PHI can (and should) be monitored, resulting in notifications of security breaches. If the patients they are concerned about have opted into the facility directory, the concerned staff members may request the patients' basic information (fact of admission, location in facility, and general condition) from the facility directory or visit the patient (if the patient is receptive) using information obtained from the facility directory. Any access available to staff members by virtue of the fact that they are staff, however, must cease at the time of transfer. Once they are no longer involved in the patient's treatment, their status is the same as any other person who is generally interested in the patient's well-being.

Are These Facebook Postings a Problem?

Kimberly is a patient care assistant at Memorial Hospital. She is also an avid Facebook user. Occasionally she posts on Facebook about her work. On Monday she posted:

"Devastating…am caring for a sweet 16-year-old girl with cancer. Cannot believe her misfortune."

On Wednesday she posted:

"My 16-year-old patient's mom and dad came to visit her from their home in Middleville, 3 hours away. They brought her some items from her room at their home so she'd feel more comfortable here."

On Friday she posted:

"My sewing group is reaching out to my 16-year-old patient. They are making a blanket for her and will deliver it to her next week."

Regarding all three posts, Memorial Hospital should have a policy in place that prohibits or restricts any workplace discussions using social media, particularly where patients are involved. In general, these posts send a message that Memorial Hospital and its workforce (Kimberly) do not value their patients' privacy. They could result in lawsuits.

These posts should also be reviewed, however, to determine if the information disclosed is PHI and, subsequently, if the posts are HIPAA violations. The first part of the PHI test (whether the posts contain individually identifiable information) is in question and will be discussed in detail. The second and third parts of the PHI three-part test are established: the information relates to the individual's present physical condition (cancer) and provision of healthcare (hospitalization) and it is held by a covered entity (Memorial Hospital).

Regarding the first part of the PHI test, HIPAA states that deidentified information is that which does not identify an individual and for which there is no reasonable basis to believe an individual could be identified based on the information provided. It provides further clarification by stating that statistics experts in statistics can determine that there is a minimal risk the information could be used to identify the patient. HIPAA also provides a list of 18 identifiers that must be removed to deidentify an individual.

- Kimberly's Monday post identifies the patient as a "16-year-old girl." It technically is not individually identifiable because the age included is below 90, and gender is not an identifier.

- Kimberly's Wednesday post identifies the parents' and patient's home as Middleville. HIPAA states that geographic units containing fewer than 20,000 people are identifiable. The population of Middleville is significant. Depending on its size, Kimberly may or may not have committed a HIPAA violation.

- Kimberly's Friday post goes a step further. Although no additional individually identifiable information is disclosed, it is implied that she has disclosed or will disclose the patient's name so her sewing group members can deliver the blanket. Even if the patient has opted into the facility directory, information in the facility directory cannot be disclosed unless the requester asks for the patient by name (which the sewing group members can only obtain from Kimberly).

Finally, the posts that are determined to be HIPAA violations may or may not be breaches. A breach is unauthorized acquisition, access, use, or disclosure of unsecured PHI (that is, it is usable, readable or decipherable to unauthorized persons). For a breach to have occurred, one of the three exceptions (unintentional acquisition, inadvertent disclosure, or situations where the recipient would not have been able to retain the information) could not have been met. Finally, Memorial Hospital must determine, through a risk assessment of each posting, whether the probability of the PHI have been compromised as a result of the violation is low. If not, then a breach has occurred. If any of the postings are determined to be breaches, the patient's parents (since she is a minor) must be notified without unreasonable delay and the breaches must be reported to HHS. Appropriate action must be taken to deal with Kimberly in all of these situations.

May a Physician's Office Leave Messages with Family Members or on Voicemail to Remind Patients of Appointments?

HIPAA allows covered entities to communicate with an individual about the individual's healthcare or payment of healthcare. This includes leaving messages with family members or on answering machines. The individual must have been notified of this activity in the covered entity's Notice of Privacy Practices. Messages must accommodate an individual's reasonable preference for a particular communication and must be limited to the minimum necessary (for example, messages left with family members should be limited to information relevant to their involvement with that care). Personal mobile phones provide an attractive alternative for leaving messages as they are less likely to be used by individuals other than the intended recipient.

A message script keeps the content consistent and limited to the minimum necessary. Examples include: "This is Jan at phone number… This is to confirm our appointment this week at…" or "Please have … call me; he asked me to contact him."

Specific rules for facilities bound by federal drug and alcohol treatment program regulations must also be considered. Programs are permitted to communicate with patients receiving services, but messages should not ever identify the program as a source. Patients who wish their family or friends to know about their treatment must sign a consent or authorization allowing disclosure to specific individuals (Thomason 2008).

Should Employees be Allowed to Access Their Own PHI Electronically?

This creates an interesting security dilemma. HIPAA allows individuals access to their own PHI except in very limited situations, and the minimum necessary requirement does not apply. If individuals already have access to electronic health records of a covered entity because they are workforce members, it is easy for them to exercise their right of access. Allowing employee access to their own information seems consistent with HIPAA's intent. However, employees (as workforce members) should only have access to information based on their job role and as necessary to carry out their duties. Allowing employees to access their own records using their job-based access rights appears to violate these minimum necessary standards. A covered entity may have a policy requiring all requests for access be in writing (this provides further controls on access and also enables the covered entity to keep records of access). Employees who access their own information without submitting requests would be in violation of the policy. Finally, allowing employees to use job-based access rights could endanger data integrity as many employees have the ability to change information as well as review it, depending on their job role. An ideal solution would be a patient portal that enables all patients (both employees and non-employees) to view their own records in a secure manner. This way, employees would have the same rights as other patients.

If covered entities have been permissive in the past regarding employee access, it may be difficult to begin prohibiting it and applying sanctions for inappropriately accessing one's own information. On the other hand, employees who are free to access their own records outside the scope of their job role may become comfortable accessing others' information (for example, friends', neighbors', and coworkers') out of curiosity, thus committing HIPAA violations.

Finally, taking away the freedom to access one's own information will eliminate the apparent discrimination that results when some employees can access their information because of existing job-based access rights while others cannot because their jobs do not grant them as much, or any, access to electronic systems (Thomason 2008).

May We Disclose a Patient's Name If He or She Has a Communicable Disease?

Most states have laws that require reporting of communicable diseases with the purpose of protecting the health of the public. In those cases, the name of a patient with a communicable disease must be reported (the law is mandatory, not permissive). State law may also be permissive, allowing the reporting to occur but not requiring it.

HIPAA allows disclosure of PHI without individual authorization if it serves one of 12 public interest and benefit purposes. Per HIPAA, a covered entity may disclose communicable disease information under one of two public and interest benefit sections: first, covered entities may disclose information as required by other laws; second, covered entities may disclose information for the purpose of public health, disease prevention, or control. Even if a state public health law appears to give a patient less privacy than what the Privacy Rule requires, it still must be followed. The Privacy Rule exempts state public health statutes from HIPAA preemption.

Medicare Conditions of Participation and state licensure rules also generally require that covered entities have infection control plans, which include identifying sources of infection and individuals who may be exposed to a communicable disease. For example, an infection control nurse may use and disclose PHI regarding a communicable disease under the healthcare operations provisions of the Privacy Rule (although the minimum necessary requirement applies to operations).

If an individual has a highly contagious disease, it is best to contact the applicable public health agency, which will notify others who may have been exposed. Even when state laws do not specifically require such disclosures, HIPAA's public interest and benefit provision regarding threats to health and safety permits disclosures by a covered entity to prevent or lessen a serious and imminent threat to the health of a person or the public. The disclosure can be made to the person in danger or an authority (such as a health department) who can lessen the threat.

Specific rules for facilities bound by federal drug and alcohol treatment program regulations must also be considered. Disclosures for public health purposes are not permitted if they identify the patient as being part of a federally protected drug and alcohol treatment program. Disclosure may be made pursuant to the patient's authorization or without identifying the patient (Thomason 2008).

Do Patients Have to Sign an Authorization to Obtain Their Own Records?

HIPAA does not require that patients sign an authorization to obtain their own records. However, state law may require a written authorization from the patient. HIPAA permits a covered entity to craft its own policy regarding this issue.

Even if no state law requires authorization, there may be practical or procedural reasons to require that individuals provide a written request even if they are the recipients of their own information. Written requests may be the only way to verify the identity of the requestor (for example, by comparing the signature to one in the patient's record) when the request is not made in person. Also, there may be a need to document the authority of a personal representative who is requesting the records of someone else. Finally, a written authorization provides additional documentation for keeping track of disclosures that were made. It should be noted that requests by individuals for their own records do not have to meet the requirements of a HIPAA-compliant authorization. Thus, a handwritten request from a patient with sufficient information to identify what they are requesting and who they are is adequate for the covered entity to release the records (Thomason 2008).

Does an Individual Have the Right to Opt out of Being Listed in a Facility Directory, Yet Demand Information Be Provided to Specific People When They Call?

HIPAA allows individuals to decide if they want to be listed in a facility directory when they are admitted to a facility. If the patient decides to be listed in the facility directory, he or she should be informed that only callers who ask for the patient by name will be given any information. Religious affiliation is also often listed with the patient's permission, in case the patient would like a visit from clergy of the patient's denomination.

The covered entity must provide the individual with the choice to restrict or prohibit some or all of these uses or disclosures. Most entities have interpreted this as giving an individual a choice to be listed in or not listed in the directory, nothing in between. "Out of the directory" means that all disclosures to visitors or callers are prohibited. Often this ban is absolute. No calls will be forwarded and no flowers delivered. If patients want visitors to know where they are, the patients themselves or their family must inform visitors. The assumption is that these patients are requesting absolute privacy.

Covered entities generally do not provide screening of visitors or of calls for patients because such an activity is too difficult to manage. Too many employees and volunteers are involved in the process of forwarding calls and directing visitors for the covered entity to ensure that patients' requests are honored. If a covered entity agreed to this screening and could not meet the agreement, it could be considered a violation of this standard of the Privacy Rule.

The restriction or prohibition of some information is usually applied to the question of clergy. The restriction is easy enough to implement; the patient need only indicate that he or she does not want to list a denomination. As clergy visiting lists are only provided based on a patient's denomination, no external clergyperson would be provided the patient's name (Thomason 2008).

Is This Gift a HIPAA Violation?

Mary was a patient at Select OB/Gyn. When she found out she was pregnant, she met with an OB nurse to discuss her diet and other prenatal issues. Mary later suffered a miscarriage. Two days after her scheduled due date, Mary received a congratulatory package of baby formula in the mail from a manufacturer. When Mary asked Select OB/Gyn about this, the privacy officer responded that Mary had been notified via the Notice of Privacy Practices that her name may be given to companies as part of Select's healthcare operations. Mary was further informed that she had signed a consent form, granting permission to Select to disclose her PHI for TPO purposes. Robin had the same experience as Mary, but Robin delivered a healthy baby boy and was thrilled to receive a package of free baby formula. Did Select OB/Gyn commit a HIPAA violation by sharing these patients' information?

HIPAA defines marketing as a communication about a product or service that encourages the recipient to purchase or use that product or service. HIPAA's general rule is that an individual's authorization must be obtained prior to using his or her PHI for marketing. There are five specific types of communications that appear to be marketing, but do not meet the definition and therefore do not require an authorization (for example, communications that describe replacements or enhancements to health plan). Two additional types of communications meet the marketing definition, but HIPAA does not require an authorization. These are face-to-face communications occurring between the covered entity and the individual, and communications concerning a promotional gift of nominal value provided by the covered entity. The sharing of Mary's and Robin's information does not fit into these exceptions.

One might argue that Select OB/Gyn's position is compelling: first, Mary was informed of the disclosure (defined as healthcare operations) via the Notice of Privacy Practices; and second, she signed a consent form granting disclosure of her PHI for TPO purposes. The problem with Select's logic, however, is that its dissemination of PHI—while described as healthcare operations—was actually marketing.

It is irrelevant that Robin was thrilled to receive a package of free baby formula. While she may not complain about it, her HIPAA rights were violated just as Mary's were.

HITECH has sought to limit efforts by covered entities and BAs to portray marketing activities as healthcare operations. HITECH expands activities defined as marketing and limits the definition of healthcare operations to stop current marketing practices and increase the numbers and types of activities for which authorization is required for use and disclosure to occur. Further, per HITECH, if Mary's and Robin's information was disclosed (with their authorization, of course) in exchange for any financial compensation (that is, their information was sold by Select OB/Gyn to the baby formula manufacturer), this fact must be clearly disclosed.

Are "White Boards" Allowed Per HIPAA?

White boards, erasable patient information boards, provide a way to communicate certain information about patients to the healthcare providers who care for them. For example, a white board might contain patient safety-related information about an individual patient such as fall precautions, transfer status, and difficulty in swallowing. This is important information for a healthcare provider to know. HIPAA repeatedly states that the intent of the Privacy Rule is not to interfere with customary and necessary communications in the healthcare of the individual. In this case, the safety of the patient comes first.

This information should be limited to the minimum necessary for the purpose, and the white board should be posted in a designated area to reduce disclosures to individuals who are not involved in the care of the patient, such as to visitors to the patient's room. Visitors may see this information on a white board posted in the patient's room, but often these visitors are family or friends who have been invited by the patient; therefore, the healthcare provider can assume the patient is comfortable with the visitors seeing the information. The patient should be informed of the right to deny access to any "well meaning, but intrusive visitors." Some providers use symbols known only to the healthcare providers to communicate the information.

A second type of white board may have multiple patients' information listed. It is used by healthcare providers to monitor the current status and location of patients in areas where the patients' status or location is frequently changing. This type of white board may be effectively used in an emergency or obstetrical department. Each facility needs to assess the use of these status boards based on certain criteria:

- Is the white board essential to the communication in the department?
- Does the white board's presence add to the safe and efficient treatment of the patients involved?
- Is the information about the patient limited to the minimum necessary for the purpose?
- Can initials be used instead of names?
- Can room numbers be used instead of names?
- Are all of the critical elements and required data listed and displayed in a manner that is useful for the healthcare providers?
- Is the white board located in the best location to reduce incidental disclosures, and is it out of the sight lines of the public?
- Finally, have other options been explored that might function just as well?

It is recommended that answers to these questions be documented by the facility. It is valuable that someone knowledgeable about HIPAA, such as the privacy officer, assess the use. Overall white board use in the facility should also be reassessed periodically to ensure the above criteria are still being met (Thomason 2008).

Can Patients Sign in for Appointments?

HIPAA allows communications to occur for treatment purposes. Its intent is not to interfere with customary and necessary communications for the care of the individual. Patients may sign their names on a waiting room list, and if another patient sees it, that is considered an incidental disclosure.

However, the healthcare provider must take reasonable precautions that the information is limited to the minimum necessary for the purpose. For example, patients should never be asked to write the reason for their visit or whether they have health insurance. Some providers have attempted to limit the disclosure by having patients sign in on a label sheet, which allows their names to be removed as soon as they are registered.

Additionally, there are specific rules for facilities bound by federal drug and alcohol treatment program regulations. They permit the disclosure of a patient's name as long it is not used in connection with the fact that the patient is receiving drug or alcohol treatment services. If a program shares a waiting room with other providers, a sign-in log would be permitted if the patient did not have to indicate he or she was there for program services (Thomason 2008).

What Can Be Done to Protect Privacy in Semiprivate Rooms?

HIPAA allows communications for treatment purposes and between healthcare providers and patients. Its intent is not to interfere with customary and necessary communications for the care of the individual. However, there are situations in which incidental disclosures cannot be reduced.

Suggestions for increasing patient privacy in semiprivate rooms include using television or radio static to muffle conversations, keeping voices as low as possible, or hanging sound muffling curtains. However, background static or low voices may also prevent the patient from hearing information needed to make critical health discussions. There is often very little space in these rooms, especially when treatment-related machines, walkers, and other treatment paraphernalia for two patients are added to the room. Sometimes, the healthcare provider does not have enough room to pull the curtain far enough to maintain privacy during discussions. Of course, the provider can ask the other patient's visitors to leave the room, so at least the visitors do not hear the discussions. As it is nearly impossible to maintain privacy in these rooms, this was one reason why incidental disclosures are not considered HIPAA violations (Thomason 2008).

What Is a Good Way to Dispose of Items, Such as Specimen Cups and IV Bags That Have PHI on Them?

HIPAA requires covered entities to take reasonable precautions to safeguard PHI used for TPO. It is critical for patient care and safety that certain items be labeled with the patient's identity. Labeling these items with identifiable information is considered a part of treatment.

When the question of shredding prescription vials as a requirement of the Privacy Rule arose, the Office for Civil Rights, in its published guidance documents, initially answered in the negative. However, shredding PHI on paper appears to be a reasonable safeguard to meet this section of the regulation. In an effort to meet this requirement, covered entities have realized that it is not only paper or electronic records that contain PHI. Other byproducts of the treatment process have individually identifiable information as well.

There are four common methods used by healthcare facilities to destroy the PHI on specimen cups, IV bags, and similar items: use permanent markers to mark out the PHI before discarding the item in the regular trash; remove the labels and place the labels in confidential trash to be shredded; place the items in biohazard trash; or place special labels over the PHI prior to disposal.

When a covered entity is deciding on a method of deidentifying these items for disposal, it is important that the choice of a safeguard be reasonable. The probability of risk of disclosure based on a person retrieving one of these identifiable items should be balanced against the cost and effort to deidentify the item. The covered entity may find that placing such items in biohazard bags is extremely expensive because of the additional cost to pay for the destruction of these items. The facility needs to consider the time it takes for a nurse to place special labels to cover the patient's name and decide whether this activity is a good use of skilled, highly-paid personnel (Thomason 2008).

Are Privacy Screens on Personal Computers (PCs) a Good Idea?

HIPAA requires covered entities to provide reasonable safeguards to prevent incidental disclosures. Incidental disclosures are considered the unintentional communications of individually identifiable information to a person who should not see or hear the information.

A privacy screen on a PC is a good option when the covered entity has employees located in areas where the public may see the contents of the screen while the screen has individually identifiable information displayed on it. Privacy screens are useful in common areas such as reception areas, admitting areas, or open nursing stations. However, HIPAA requires that covered entities make reasonable efforts to meet this standard. Requiring these screens on all PCs, even in areas restricted from the public, may be expensive and not reasonable.

Other options are password protected screensavers set to activate after a period of time, standard display mounting equipment that can minimize exposure of PHI, or doors to hide the monitor when not actively in use (Thomason 2008).

Is It Okay to Communicate Health Information Using Messaging Service Software?

HIPAA requires that a covered entity must provide reasonable safeguards to protect individually identifiable information. The Security Rule would require that the risks to security and privacy be assessed with the use of any software product used by the covered entity.

Setting aside other security considerations, the main threat to privacy in using messaging service software is that PHI can be transmitted outside of the covered entity using messaging services. Not only may an inappropriate disclosure be made, but transmitting messages using this software is not very secure and can be easily breached. It is possible to install monitoring and filtering software, but this is difficult and certainly not something a covered entity can depend on to adequately protect the covered entity from inappropriate disclosures. Managers at the department level can monitor workforce use. However, this may not be a practical approach.

The covered entity has the responsibility to implement policies and procedures to address the disclosure of PHI. Limitations on use or nonuse of this type of software should be addressed in policies about secure transmission of PHI, as well as in policies outlining when disclosure of PHI is permitted. The covered entity also has the responsibility to educate the workforce on those policies and to sanction a member of the workforce should they violate the policy or regulations regarding the disclosure of PHI.

If the covered entity determines that the use of messaging services is a high risk to the privacy and security of the institution, and there is difficulty monitoring its use, they should not permit its use by the workforce (Thomason 2008).

Should a Physician Be Able to Access an Electronic Health Record at Home?

HIPAA permits healthcare providers to access PHI for treatment purposes. However, the Security Rule requires a covered entity to provide reasonable safeguards to protect the information. Further, the Security Rule requires a covered entity to

- Ensure the confidentiality, integrity, and availability of all electronic PHI the covered entity creates, receives, maintains, or transmits
- Protect against any reasonably anticipated threats or hazards to the security or integrity of such information

- Protect against any reasonably anticipated uses or disclosures of such information not permitted or required
- Ensure compliance by its workforce

These requirements are not easy to meet when the access is from an unsecured location. In addition, if the physician has access and can print or copy the information, it further increases the possibility of a violation of the regulations.

Proper technology can mitigate some of the risks. Physicians can gain access via a dedicated portal on a secure gateway or have Virtual Private Network (VPN) access. This goes a long way to protect the security of the delivery method. These portals can be configured so that any printing will not include the header information containing the identity of the patient. The covered entity is responsible for the electronic record and must evaluate the benefits to patient treatment and convenience to the physician against the risks to patient privacy.

Finally, it is worth noting that if the physician is a separate covered entity, the physician has the responsibility to meet the same HIPAA privacy and security standards as the covered entity that creates and maintains the records. In this circumstance, the covered entity that provides the electronic access may require a physician to sign an agreement that, in return for the privilege of accessing the health record from home, he or she will provide reasonable safeguards to protect the information (Thomason 2008).

Does HIPAA Define Where a Fax Machine Should Be Placed in a Facility?

HIPAA does not specify where machines containing or transmitting PHI should be located. A covered entity must safeguard PHI and take reasonable steps to do so. The Security Rule does not apply to faxed information, as facsimiles are generally not considered electronic PHI unless the fax is computer to computer. In order to safeguard PHI, a covered entity should use common sense and the best security practices to determine where to place fax machines or copiers that receive confidential faxes.

Fax machines should be placed where they are convenient for staff, but not where the information can be viewed or retrieved by unauthorized persons. Faxed material should not be left unattended for long periods of time. A fax machine should be in a secure area. If used by several departments, unique mailboxes should be designated for each department so that the faxes can be stored but not printed until an authorized person does so.

A covered entity should provide guidelines for its workforce on when faxing information is permitted, as the risk of accidental disclosure is greater when using a fax than when using mail. The outgoing fax should include a cover sheet that identifies the accompanying information as confidential and contains a number to call should the fax be misdirected. Automatic fax systems should be routinely audited to ensure that the numbers are accurate and numbers should be confirmed before information is sent. Information should be faxed only when necessary, and highly sensitive information (for example, HIV or AIDS information) should not be faxed if possible. Faxed information should also be encrypted during transit (Thomason 2008).

What Should We Do When a Laptop with Protected Health Information Is Stolen or Lost?

If a laptop or storage media that contains protected heath information is lost or stolen, the covered entity must review the risks to individuals whose information was contained in the laptop.

The covered entity should have established an incident response team or process to call upon in this situation, as required by the HIPAA Security Rule. These teams often include individuals with expertise in information systems, risk management, law and regulations, public relations, and human resources. The covered entity must first attempt to determine the information that was contained on the laptop. Some of the content may be found by examining backups made by the laptop user to internal servers, reviewing system activity logs, stored queries, and use of e-mail by the user. The user of the laptop should be interviewed to determine if there was a password protecting the laptop, if the data was encrypted, the circumstances of the theft, and what the person recalls as being stored on the laptop.

The assessment of risk to the individuals whose information is contained on the laptop depends on the degree and type of information that was stored on the laptop that is individually identifiable. If the information contains sensitive diagnosis information, or if the information includes social security numbers, credit card numbers, or PINs, the risk to the individuals becomes significant (for example, a person may steal a laptop computer for the malicious purpose of publishing the information it contains or committing identity theft).

If the names of individuals whose information is contained in the stolen laptop can be identified by the covered entity, the theft of the laptop should be included in information provided for the accounting of disclosures. Therefore, if an individual requests an accounting of disclosures, the information would be available to the individual (Thomason 2008).

Per HITECH, the covered entity is required to notify the affected individuals if it determines that a breach occurred. Whether or not the data was encrypted (that is, whether it was unsecured) will be significant in making this determination. The covered entity must also take other steps that would mitigate any harmful effect the covered entity knows about that may have resulted. It has become common practice to offer credit monitoring services to individuals when there has been a breach of information that could be used for identity theft.

Appendix D

CHECK YOUR UNDERSTANDING ANSWER KEY

Chapter 1

Check Your Understanding 1.1
1. False
2. True
3. False
4. True
5. True

Check Your Understanding 1.2
1. False
2. True
3. True
4. False
5. False

Chapter 2

Check Your Understanding 2.1
1. False
2. False
3. False
4. False
5. False

Check Your Understanding 2.2
1. True
2. True
3. False
4. True
5. True

Chapter 3

Check Your Understanding 3.1
1. False
2. False
3. False
4. True
5. True

Check Your Understanding 3.2
1. True
2. True
3. True
4. True
5. False

Check Your Understanding 3.3
1. False
2. True
3. False
4. False
5. True

Chapter 4

Check Your Understanding 4.1
1. True
2. False
3. True
4. False
5. True

Check Your Understanding 4.2
1. True
2. True
3. False
4. False
5. False

Check Your Understanding 4.3

1. True
2. True
3. True
4. True
5. True

Chapter 5

Check Your Understanding 5.1

1. True
2. False
3. True
4. False
5. False

Check Your Understanding 5.2

1. True
2. True
3. False
4. False
5. True

Chapter 6

Check Your Understanding 6.1

1. False
2. False
3. True
4. True
5. True

Check Your Understanding 6.2

1. True
2. False
3. False
4. True
5. True

Glossary

Access: (1) The ability of a subject to view, change, or communicate with an object in a computer system; (2) One of the rights protected by the Privacy Rule; an individual has a right of access to inspect and obtain a copy of his or her own PHI that is contained in a designated record set, such as a health record

Access report: Individual right proposed by the Department of Health and Human Services on May 31, 2011 that would enable individuals to find out who has accessed their electronic PHI, including persons who accessed it as part of their routine work; the right would be applicable to EHRs and ePHI in a designated record set

Account lockout: Prohibited access to an electronic account after an established number of attempts have been made

Accounting of disclosures: HIPAA requirement to list, upon patient request, all disclosures that meet the criteria. Currently, this does not require accounting for disclosures for Treatment, Payment, and healthcare Operations (TPO), but under ARRA this changes to include these disclosures for EHRs; awaiting final regulations

Accreditation: (1) A voluntary process of institutional or organizational review in which a quasi-independent body created for this purpose periodically evaluates the quality of the entity's work against preestablished written criteria; (2) A determination by an accrediting body that an eligible organization, network, program, group, or individual complies with applicable standards; (3) The act of granting approval to a healthcare organization based on whether the organization has met a set of voluntary standards developed by an accreditation agency

Accreditation Association for Ambulatory Health Care (AAAHC): A professional organization that offers accreditation programs for ambulatory and outpatient organizations such as single-specialty and multispecialty group practices, ambulatory surgery centers, college or university health services, and community health centers

Addressable specifications: The implementation specifications of the HIPAA Security Rule that are designated "addressable" rather than "required"; to be in compliance with the Rule, the covered entity must implement the specification as written, implement an alternative, or document that the risk for which the addressable implementation specification was provided either does not exist in the organization, or exists with a negligible probability of occurrence

Administrative Procedure Act (APA): A federal statute that imposes procedural uniformity on federal administrative agencies and governs how they may propose and establish rules (regulations)

Administrative rule: A law created by an administrative agency that provides greater detail than a statute so the statute can be implemented or carried out; also referred to as a regulation

Administrative safeguards: A set of nine standards defined by the HIPAA Security Rule. Administrative actions such as policies and procedures and documentation retention to manage the selection, development, implementation, and maintenance of security measures to protect electronic protected health information and manage the conduct of the covered entity's or business associate's workforce in relation to the protection of that information

Administrative simplification: A term referring to the HIPAA provisions which include standards for transactions and code sets that are used to exchange health data, standard identifiers for use on transactions, and privacy and security standards to protect personal health information. HIPAA included these administrative simplification provisions in order to improve the efficiency and effectiveness of the healthcare system

Affiliated covered entity: Legally-separate covered entities, affiliated by common ownership or control; for purposes of the Privacy Rule, these legally separate entities may refer to themselves as a single covered entity

Altered authorization: An authorization in which one or more of HIPAA's authorization requirements related to a research study have been changed per institutional review board or privacy board approval

Amendment: Alteration of health information by modification, correction, addition, or deletion

American Health Information Management Association (AHIMA) Code of Ethics: A document that provides guidance to members of the health information profession regarding ethical principles; as evidence of an AHIMA-credentialed individual's professional values and principles; it does not have the force and effect of law, but violation of the Code of Ethics can result in disciplinary action including revocation of AHIMA credentials

American National Standards Institute (ANSI): An organization that governs standards in many aspects of public and private business; developer of the Health Information Technology Standards Panel

American Osteopathic Association (AOA): The professional association of osteopathic physicians, surgeons, and graduates of approved colleges of osteopathic medicine that inspects and accredits osteopathic colleges and hospitals

American Recovery and Reinvestment Act (ARRA) of 2009: An economic stimulus package enacted by the 111th United States Congress in February 2009; signed into law by President Obama on February 17th, 2009; an unprecedented effort to jumpstart the economy, create/save millions of jobs, and put a down payment on addressing long-neglected challenges; an extraordinary response to a crisis unlike any since the Great Depression and includes measures to modernize our nation's infrastructure, enhance energy independence, expand educational opportunities, preserve and improve affordable health care, provide tax relief, and protect those in greatest need

Antivirus software packages: Computer programs that search for malicious software (malware) that can damage an information system; anti-virus software packages prevent, detect or remove viruses

Audit controls: The mechanisms that record and examine activity in information systems

Audit log: A chronological record of electronic system(s) activities that enables the reconstruction, review, and examination of the sequence of events surrounding or leading to each event and/or transaction from its beginning to end. Includes who performed what event and when it occurred

Audit trail: (1) A chronological set of computerized records that provides evidence of information system activity (log-ins and log-outs, file accesses) used to determine security violations; (2) A record that shows who has accessed a computer system, when it was accessed, and what operations were performed

Authentication: (1) The process of identifying the source of health record entries by attaching a handwritten signature, the author's initials, or an electronic signature; (2) Proof of authorship that ensures, as much as possible, that log-ins and messages from a user originate from an authorized source

Authorization: (1) The granting of permission to disclose confidential information; as defined in terms of the HIPAA privacy rule, an individual's formal, written permission to use or disclose his or her personally identifiable health information for purposes other than treatment, payment, or healthcare operations; (2) A patient's consent to the disclosure of protected health information (PHI); the form by which a patient gives consent to release of information

Breach: A violation of a legal duty or wrongful conduct that serves as the basis for a civil remedy

Breach notification: HITECH Act Rule that requires both HIPAA-covered entities and business associates to identify unsecured PHI breaches and notify the involved parties of the breach

"Break the glass": A computer system capability that allows an individual who otherwise does not have access privileges to ePHI to access it through an alternative method in limited, necessary situations such as patient care emergencies

Business associate (BA): (1) According to the HIPAA privacy rule, an individual (or group) who is not a member of a covered entity's workforce but who helps the covered entity in the performance of various functions involving the use or disclosure of individually identifiable health information or disclosure of individually identifiable health information; (2) A person or organization other than a member of a covered entity's workforce that performs functions or activities on behalf of or affecting a covered entity that involve the use or disclosure of individually identifiable health information

Business associate agreement (BAA): A written and signed contract that allows covered entities to lawfully disclose protected health information to business associates such as consultants, billing companies, accounting firms, or others that may perform services for the provider, provided that the business associate agrees to abide by the provider's requirements to protect the information's security and confidentiality

Business continuity plan: A program that incorporates policies and procedures for continuing business operations during a computer system shutdown

Centers for Medicare and Medicaid Services (CMS): The division of the Department of Health and Human Services that is responsible for developing healthcare policy in the United States and for administering the Medicare program and the federal portion of the Medicaid program and maintaining the procedure portion of the International Classification of Diseases, ninth revision, Clinical Modification (ICD-9-CM); called the Health Care Financing Administration (HCFA) prior to 2001

Certification: (1) The process by which a duly authorized body evaluates and recognizes an individual, institution, or educational program as meeting predetermined requirements; (2) An evaluation performed to establish the extent to which a particular computer system, network design, or application implementation meets a prespecified set of requirements

Certification Commission for Health Information Technology (CCHIT): An independent, voluntary, private-sector initiative organized as a limited liability corporation that has been awarded a contract by the U.S. Department of Health and Human Services (HHS) to develop, create prototypes for, and evaluate the certification criteria and inspection process for electronic health record products (EHRs)

Child Abuse Prevention and Treatment Act (CAPTA) of 1996: A federal child abuse and neglect reporting statute that is used as a model for many state child abuse and neglect statutes

Clinical Laboratory Improvements Amendments (CLIA) of 1988: Passed in 1988, the amendment established quality standards for all laboratory testing to ensure the accuracy, reliability, and timeliness of patient test results regardless of where the test is

Code of Federal Regulations (CFR): The official collection of legislative and regulatory guidelines mandated by final rules published in the *Federal Register*

Commission on Accreditation of Rehabilitation Facilities (CARF): An accreditation body that focuses on health and human service providers

Comprehensive Alcohol Abuse and Alcoholism Prevention, Treatment, and Rehabilitation Act of 1970: A federal statute that specifically protects information related to drug or other substance abuse

Compound authorizations: Authorizations that combine informed consent, often for participation in research activities, with an authorization to use or disclose one's PHI; generally limited under HIPAA

Conditioned authorizations: Authorizations that make treatment, payment, and health plan enrollment or benefit eligibility contingent on the signing of the authorization; generally prohibited by HIPAA

Conditions of Participation (CoP): The administrative and operational guidelines and regulations under which facilities are allowed to take part in the Medicare and Medicaid programs; published by the Centers for Medicare and Medicaid Services, a federal agency under the Department of Health and Human Services

Confidential communications: As defined by HIPAA, a request that PHI be routed to an alternative location or by an alternative method

Consent: (1) A patient's acknowledgement that he or she understands a proposed intervention, including that intervention's risks, benefits, and alternatives; (2) The document signed by the patient that indicates agreement that protected health information (PHI) can be disclosed

Context-based access control (CBAC): An access control system which limits users to accessing information not only in accordance with their identity and role, but to the location and time in which they are accessing the information

Contingency plan: (1) Documentation of the process for responding to a system emergency, including the performance of backups, the line-up of critical alternative facilities to facilitate continuity of operations, and the process of recovering from a disaster; (2) A recovery plan in the event of a power failure, disaster, or other emergency that limits or eliminates access to facilities and electronic protected personal health information (ePHI)

Control analysis: The fourth step in risk analysis; it looks at ways that an organization controls its vulnerabilities to threats with the goal of eliminating or at least reducing the likelihood that a threat will successfully take advantage of a vulnerability

Control recommendations: The eighth step in risk analysis; assesses how an organization can deal with a vulnerability when it does not have a control in place

Core operations: Functions the organization decides must continue despite an event

Covered entity: A health plan, healthcare clearinghouse, or a healthcare provider that transmits individually identifiable health information in electronic form

Creditor: Defined by the Fair and Accurate Credit Transaction Act (FACTA) as "anyone who regularly, and in the ordinary course of business, obtains or uses consumer reports in connection with a credit transaction; furnishes information to consumer reporting agencies in connection with a credit transaction; or advances funds to, or on behalf of, someone, except for funds for expenses incidental to a service provided by the creditor to that person;" this definition is used to determine applicability to the Red Flags Rule

Cryptography: (1) The art of keeping data secret through the use of mathematical or logical functions that transform intelligible data into seemingly unintelligible data and back again; (2) The study of encryption and decryption techniques

Data backup: A plan that ensures the recovery of information that has been lost or becomes inaccessible

Data recovery: The retrieval of information that has been lost due to an event

Data use agreement: A document that sets the parameters for permitted uses and disclosures by the recipient of the limited data set

Decryption: Restoration of scrambled or encoded data to meaningful, readable data

Deidentified information: Health information from which all names and other identifying descriptors have been removed to protect the privacy of the patients, family members, and healthcare providers who were involved in the case

Designated record set (DRS): A group of records maintained by or for a covered entity that may include patient medical and billing records; the enrollment, payment, claims adjudication, and cases or medical management record systems maintained by or for a health plan; or information used, in whole or in part, to make patient care-related decisions

Direct final rule: A type of final administrative rule that is published without being preceded by a notice of proposed rulemaking; it is published with a statement that it will become effective on an established date unless adverse comments are received; generally applicable to noncontroversial rules

Disaster recovery plan: The document that defines the resources, actions, tasks, and data required to manage the businesses recovery process in the event of a business interruption

Disclosure: The act of making information known; in the health information management context, the release of confidential health information about an identifiable person to another person or entity

Drug Abuse Prevention, Treatment, and Rehabilitation Act of 1972: A federal statute that specifically protects information related to drug or other substance abuse

Electronic Healthcare Network Accreditation Commission (EHNAC): An organization that accredits electronic health networks by assessing them against electronic transaction standards

Electronic protected health information (ePHI): Under HIPAA, all individually identifiable information that is created or received electronically by a healthcare provider or any other entity subject to HIPAA requirements

E-mail: The electronic exchange of information using a computer network

Emergency mode of operations: A plan that defines the processes and controls that will be followed until the operations are fully restored

Encryption: The process of transforming text into an unintelligible string of characters that can be transmitted via communications media with a high degree of security and then decrypted when it reaches a secure destination

Enforcement Rule: A rule that created standardized procedures and substantive requirements for investigating complaints and imposing civil monetary penalties (CMPs) for HIPAA violations, as well as a uniform compliance and enforcement mechanism that addresses all of the Administrative Simplification regulations, including privacy, security, and transactions and code sets

Entity authentication: The corroboration that an entity is who it claims to be

External threats: Threats to information privacy and security that originate outside an organization

Facility directory: A directory of patients being treated in a healthcare facility

Facsimile (fax): A machine that allows the remote transmission of text and graphics through telephone lines or a communication sent via this method

Fair and Accurate Credit Transaction Act (FACTA): Federal statute passed in 2003 that contains provisions and requirements to reduce identity theft

Federal Register: The daily publication of the US Government Printing Office that reports all changes in regulations and federally mandated standards

Final rule: An administrative rule that is published after public comments have been considered in response to a prior proposed rule; a final rule has the full force and effect of law

Firewall: A computer system or a combination of systems that provides a security barrier or supports an access control policy between two networks or between a network and any other traffic outside the network

Flexible: A characteristic of the HIPAA Security Rule that allows a covered entity to use any security measures that allow it to reasonably and appropriately implement the Security Rule's standards and implementation specifications

Formal rulemaking: A method by which federal administrative agencies may create administrative rules; includes a trial-type hearing and has limited applicability in federal rulemaking

Freedom of Information Act (FOIA) of 1967: The federal law, applicable only to federal agencies, through which individuals can seek access to information without the authorization of the person to whom the information applies

Full disk encryption: A process that signifies all data on a disk is encrypted

Fundraising: An activity that financially benefits a covered entity; is limited by HIPAA and HITECH if PHI is used

General support systems: Any system that stores or processes ePHI

Genetic Information Nondiscrimination Act (GINA): A 2008 federal statute that prohibits the use of genetic information to determine health insurance eligibility and employment. HIPAA requirements relative to GINA were included in the January 2013 final rule.

Government Accountability Office (GAO): An independent agency that works on behalf of Congress to audit how the federal government spends taxpayer dollars; provides feedback before final administrative rules take effect

Harm threshold: Per the August 2009 Interim Final Rule, a barometer applied by covered entities and business associates to determine if a HIPAA violation is a security breach. This standard was replaced in the January 2013 final rule with the following: An impermissible use or disclosure of PHI is presumed to be a breach unless the covered entity or business associate demonstrates low probability of the PHI having been compromised

Health Information Exchange (HIE): The exchange of health information electronically between providers and others with the same level of interoperability, such as labs and pharmacies

Health Information Technology for Economic and Clinical Health (HITECH) Act: The part of ARRA that is meant to increase the momentum of developing and implementing the EHR by 2014

Health Insurance Portability and Accountability Act (HIPAA) of 1996: The federal legislation enacted to provide continuity of health coverage, control fraud and abuse in healthcare, reduce healthcare costs, and guarantee the security and privacy of health information; limits exclusion for preexisting medical conditions, prohibits discrimination against employees and dependents based on health status, guarantees availability of health insurance to small employers, and guarantees renewability of insurance to all employees regardless of size; requires covered entities (most healthcare providers and organizations) to transmit healthcare claims in a specific format; develop, implement, and comply with the standards of the Privacy Rule and the Security Rule, and mandates that covered entities apply for and utilize national identifiers in HIPAA transactions

Health plan: An entity that provides or pays the cost of medical care on behalf of enrolled individuals; includes group health plans, health insurance issuers, health maintenance organizations, and other welfare benefit plans such as Medicare, Medicaid, CHAMPUS, and Indian Health Services

Healthcare clearinghouse: As defined under HIPAA, a public or private entity (such as a billing service, repricing company, community health management information system, or community health information system, or a value-added network) that either processes or facilitates the processing of health information received from another entity in a nonstandard format or containing nonstandard data content into standard data elements or standard transactions; or receives a standard transaction from another entity and processes or facilitates the processing of health information into nonstandard format or nonstandard data content for the receiving entity

Healthcare Effectiveness and Data Information Set (HEDIS): A tool offered by the National Committee for Quality Assurance (NCQA) that measures the quality of health plan performance relating to care and service

Healthcare Facilities Accreditation Program (HFAP): An accreditation program managed by the American Osteopathic Association that offers services to a number of healthcare facilities and services, including laboratories, ambulatory care clinics, ambulatory surgery centers, behavioral health and substance abuse treatment facilities, physical rehabilitation facilities, acute care hospitals, critical access hospitals, and hospitals providing postdoctoral training for osteopathic physicians

Healthcare operations: One of three collective functions (the other two being treatment and payment) necessary to successfully conduct business; some of HIPAA's requirements (including patient authorization) are removed or relaxed when an individual's PHI is needed to carry out a healthcare operation function; includes quality improvement, case management, review of healthcare professionals' qualifications, insurance contracting, legal and auditing functions, and customer service

Certain activities undertaken by or on behalf of, a covered entity, including: conducting quality assessment and improvement activities; reviewing the competence or qualifications of health care professionals, underwriting, premium rating, and other activities relating to the creation; renewal or replacement of a contract of health insurance or health benefits; conducting or arranging for medical review, legal services, and auditing functions; business planning and development; and business management and general administrative activities of the entity

Healthcare provider: A provider of diagnostic, medical, and surgical care as well as the services or supplies related to the health of an individual and any other person or organization that issues reimbursement claims or is paid for healthcare in the normal course of business. A provider is legally responsible for the patient's diagnosis and treatment

HIPAA Privacy Rule: The federal regulations created to implement the privacy requirements of the simplification subtitle of the Health Insurance Portability and Accountability Act of 1996; effective in 2003; afforded patients certain rights to and about their protected health information

HIPAA Security Rule: The federal regulations created to implement the security requirements of the Health Insurance Portability and Accountability Act of 1996

Hybrid entity: An entity that performs both covered and noncovered functions under the Privacy Rule; for example, a university that educates students and maintains student educational records is not covered by the Privacy Rule; however, the same university that operates a medical center is covered by the Privacy Rule as it meets the definition of "healthcare provider"

Hybrid health record: A combination of paper and electronic records; a health record that includes both paper and electronic elements

Impact analysis: A collective term used to refer to any study that determines the benefit of a proposed project, including cost-benefit analysis, return on investment, benefits realization study, or qualitative benefit study

Implementation specifications: Descriptions that define how HIPAA standards are to be implemented

In loco parentis: In the place of a parent; refers to individuals other than parents who possess the legal right to make decisions on behalf of minors

Incidental uses and disclosures: Uses and disclosures that occur as part of doing business; per HIPAA, these uses and disclosures do not require patient authorization

Individual: According to the HIPAA privacy rule, a person who is the subject of protected health information

Informal rulemaking: A method by which federal administrative agencies may create administrative rules; includes rule publication and a notice and comment

Institutional Review Board (IRB): An administrative body that provides review, oversight, guidance, and approval for research projects carried out by employees serving as researchers, regardless of the location of the research (such as a university or private research agency); responsible for protecting the rights and welfare of the human subjects involved in the research; IRB oversight is mandatory for federally funded research projects

Integrity: (1) The state of being whole or unimpaired; (2) The ability of data to maintain its structure and attributes, including protection against modification or corruption during transmission, storage, or at rest. Maintenance of data integrity is a key aspect of data quality management and security

Interim final rule: A type of final administrative rule that is published without being preceded by a notice of proposed rulemaking; it must offer a post-promulgation opportunity for public comments; based on comments, it may be confirmed as the final rule or reissued as a revised final rule

Internal threats: Threats to information privacy and security that originate within an organization

Intrusion detection systems: Software that analyze network traffic, sending an alarm if they detect potentially inappropriate attempts to access a network or particular account; require human intervention to monitor alarms and determine their validity

Intrusion prevention systems: Software that identify inappropriate electronic traffic and block its passage in a mechanism similar to a firewall; require human intervention to monitor alarms and determine their validity

Invalid log-on attempt: Use of an incorrect user name or password to enter a network or particular account

Joint Commission: A private, voluntary, not-for-profit organization that evaluates and accredits hospitals and other healthcare organizations on the basis of predefined performance standards; formerly known as The Joint Commission on Accreditation of Healthcare Organizations or JCAHO

Legal health record: Documents and data elements that a healthcare provider may include in response to legally permissible requests for patient information

Likelihood determination: The fifth step in a risk analysis; once an organization identifies events that it might reasonably expect, they are categorized based on the likelihood or probability that they will exploit the organization's vulnerabilities

Limited data set: PHI that excludes direct identifiers of the individual, the individual's relatives, employers, or household members but still does not deidentify the information

Major applications: Applications that are critical to the organization or that store PHI

Major rule: An administrative rule that must be submitted to the Federal Office of Management and Budget for analysis due to estimated costs exceeding $100 million

Marketing: The process of issuing a communication about a product or service with the purpose of encouraging recipients of the communication to purchase or use the product or service

Meaningful use: A regulation that was issued by the Centers for Medicare and Medicaid Services (CMS) on July 28, 2010 outlining an incentive program for professionals (EPs), eligible hospitals and critical access hospitals (CAHs) participating in Medicare and Medicaid programs that adopt and successfully demonstrate meaningful use of certified electronic health record (EHR) technology

Medical identity theft: A subset of identity theft, it involves "the inappropriate or unauthorized misrepresentation of one's identity, generally without the individual's knowledge or permission, to (1) obtain medical services or goods, or (2) obtain money by falsifying claims for medical services and falsifying medical records to support those claims"

Metadata: Descriptive data that characterize other data to create a clearer understanding of their meaning and to achieve greater reliability and quality of information. Metadata consist of both indexing terms and attributes. Data about data: for example, creation date, date sent, date received, last access date, last modification data

Minimum necessary: A stipulation of the HIPAA privacy rule that requires healthcare facilities and other covered entities to make reasonable efforts to limit the patient-identifiable information they disclose to the least amount required to accomplish the intended purpose for which the information was requested

Mitigation: The Privacy Rule (45 CFR 164.530(f)) requires covered entities to lessen, as much as possible, harmful effects that result from the wrongful use and disclosure of protected health information; possible courses of action may include an apology; disciplinary action against the responsible employee or employees (although such results will not be able to be shared with the wronged individual); repair of the process that resulted in the breach; payment of a bill or financial loss that resulted from the infraction; or gestures of goodwill and good public relations, such as a gift certificate, that may assuage the individual

National Center for Health Statistics (NCHS): The federal agency responsible for collecting and disseminating information on health services utilization and the health status of the population in the United States; developed the clinical modification to the International Classification of Diseases, Ninth Revision (ICD-9) and is responsible for updating the diagnosis portion of the ICD-9-CM

National Committee for Quality Assurance (NCQA): A private not-for-profit accreditation organization whose mission is to evaluate and report on the quality of managed care organizations in the United States

National Institute of Standards and Technology (NIST): An agency of the U.S. Department of Commerce, was founded in 1901 as the nation's first federal physical science research laboratory

National Voluntary Laboratory Accreditation Program (NVLAP): The ONC-designated approved accreditor (ONC-AA) that accredits organizations to serve as accredited testing laboratories and to test EHR technology

Notice of Privacy Practices (NPP): A statement (mandated by the HIPAA privacy rule) issued by a healthcare organization that informs individuals of the uses and disclosures of patient-identifiable health information that may be made by the organization, as well as the individual's rights and the organization's legal duties with respect to that information

Notice of Proposed Rulemaking (NPRM): Notice published in the *Federal Register* calling for public comment on its policy; the public at large has a specified time period to submit comments

Office for Civil Rights (OCR): Department in HHS responsible for enforcing civil rights laws that prohibit discrimination on the basis of race, color, national origin, disability, age, sex, and religion by health care and human services entities over which OCR has jurisdiction, such as state and local social and health services agencies; and hospitals, clinics, nursing homes or other entities receiving Federal Financial Assistance from HHS. This office also has the authority to ensure and enforce the HIPAA Privacy and Security Rules; OCR is responsible for investigating all alleged violations of the Privacy and Security Rules

Office of Management and Budget (OMB): The core mission of OMB is to serve the President of the United States in implementing his vision across the Executive Branch. OMB is the largest component of the Executive Office of the President. It reports directly to the President and reviews administrative rules for consistency with presidential policies and budgetary priorities

Office of the National Coordinator for Health Information Technology (ONC): The principal federal entity charged with coordination of nationwide efforts to implement and use the most advanced health information technology and the electronic exchange of health information. The position of National Coordinator was created in 2004, through an Executive Order, and legislatively mandated in the Health Information Technology for Economic and Clinical Health Act (HITECH Act) of 2009

Office of the National Coordinator for Health Information Technology-Approved Accreditor (ONC-AA): An organization designated by the Office of the National Coordinator for Health Information Technology to accredit organizations to test EHR technology

Office of the National Coordinator for Health Information Technology-Authorized Certification Body (ONC-ACB): An organization authorized by the Office of the National Coordinator for Health Information Technology to certify EHR technology; the permanent ONC-ACB program replaces the temporary ONC-ATCB program

Office of the National Coordinator for Health Information Technology-Authorized Testing and Certification Body (ONC-ATCB): An organization authorized by the Office of the National Coordinator for Health Information Technology (ONC) to test and certify EHR technology under the temporary ONC-ATCB program that was created to ensure providers had certified EHRs in place

Organized healthcare arrangement: An agreement characterized by more than one covered entity who share PHI to manage and benefit their common enterprise and are recognized by the public as a single entity

Parens patriae: Authority to act on citizens' behalf, given to state Attorneys General via HITECH to bring civil actions in federal district court on behalf of individuals believed to have been negatively affected by HIPAA violations

Patient portal: An electronic repository of information about an individual, which the individual can access via the Internet. It is often hosted and controlled by a provider or payer; in any case, it is not controlled by the individual

Payment: One of three collective functions (the other two being treatment and healthcare operations) necessary to successfully conduct business; some of HIPAA's requirements (including patient authorization) are removed or relaxed when an individual's PHI is needed to carry out a payment function; includes providers' activities to obtain reimbursement for care or services provided and health plans' activities to obtain premiums

Person authentication: A process, required by the HIPAA Security Rule, that verifies a person is who he says he is in order to prevent unauthorized users from accessing ePHI

Personal Health Record (PHR): An electronic or paper health record maintained and updated by an individual for himself or herself; a tool that an individual can use to collect, track, and share past and current information about their health or the health of someone in their care

Personal Health Record portal: An electronic repository of information about a patient that allows the patient to create and control the content of his own personal health record; is accessed through the Internet

Personal Health Record vendor: An entity that sets up and maintains a website where individuals can store their health information in an online repository; per HITECH, personal health record vendors may be business associates and therefore subject to breach notification requirements and penalties

Personal representative: Per HIPAA, a person who is treated the same as the patient with regard to the use and disclosure of the patient's PHI

Physical safeguards: Measures such as locking doors to safeguard data and various media from unauthorized access and exposures; a set of four standards defined by the HIPAA Security Rule including facility access controls, workstation use, workstation security, and device and media controls

Preemption: In law, the principle that one statute supercedes or is applied over another statute (for example, the federal HIPAA privacy provisions trump the same or similar state law except when state law is more stringent)

Privacy: The quality or state of being hidden from, or undisturbed by, the observation or activities of other persons, or freedom from unauthorized intrusion; in healthcare-related contexts, the right of a patient to control disclosure of protected health information

Privacy Act of 1974: A law that requires federal agencies to safeguard personally identifiable records and provides individuals with certain privacy rights

Privacy board: A group formed by a HIPAA-covered entity to review research studies where authorization waivers are requested and to ensure the HIPAA privacy rights of research subjects

Privacy officer: A position mandated under the HIPAA Privacy Rule—covered entities must designate an individual to be responsible for developing and implementing privacy policies and procedures

Private key infrastructure: Also called symmetric or single-key encryption; occurs where both the sending and receiving computers use software that assigns a secret code, or key; this encryption is less secure than public key encryption because the same key is transmitted with the data after the sending computer codes (scrambles) the data so the receiving computer can decode (unscramble) the data

Promulgation: The formal declaration of an administrative law (rule)

Proposed rule: The first draft of an administrative rule; it may be either a new rule or a proposed change to an existing rule

Protected health information (PHI): Individually identifiable health information, transmitted electronically or maintained in any other form, that is created, maintained, received, or transmitted by a healthcare provider or any other entity subject to HIPAA requirements

Psychotherapy notes: Notes recorded in any medium by a mental health professional to document or analyze the contents of conversations between therapists and clients during private or group counseling sessions

Public key infrastructure: Also called asymmetric encryption; uses two keys to encrypt and transmit a message; the sending computer uses a private key to code (scramble) the message and a public key is given to the receiving computer to decode (unscramble) the message

Record locator service (RLS): A service that indicates where a given patient may have health information, using probability equations

Red flags: Suspicious documents, information, or behaviors that indicate the possibility of identity theft

Red Flags Rule: A set of FTC regulations that requires certain entities to develop and implement identity theft prevention programs

Regional Health Information Organization (RHIO): A health information organization that brings together health care stakeholders within a defined geographic area and governs health information exchange among them for the purpose of improving health and care in the community

Request: To ask for access to PHI

Required specifications: The implementation specifications of the HIPAA Security Rule that are designated "required" rather than "addressable"; required standards must be present for the covered entity to be in compliance

Residual risks: Risks that continue to exist even after the organization has applied safeguards and controls

Restriction request: As defined by HIPAA, an individual's right regarding limitations on uses and disclosures of PHI for carrying out treatment, payment, and operations

Retaliation and waiver: Rights protected under the Privacy Rule; to ensure the integrity of individuals' right to complain about alleged Privacy Rule violations, covered entities are expressly prohibited from retaliating against anyone who exercises his rights under the Privacy Rule, assists in an investigation by the HHS or other appropriate investigative authority, or opposes an act or practice that the person believes is a violation of the Privacy Rule and individuals cannot be required to waive the rights that they hold under the Privacy Rule in order to obtain treatment, payment, or enrollment or benefits eligibility

Risk determination: The seventh step of risk analysis; this step considers how likely is it that a particular threat will actually occur and, if it does occur, how great its impact or severity will be and also quantifies an organization's threats, enabling it to both prioritize its risks and appropriately allocate its limited resources (namely, people, time, and money) accordingly

Risk management: A comprehensive program of activities intended to minimize the potential for injuries to occur in a facility and to anticipate and respond to ensuring liabilities for those injuries that do occur. The processes in place to identify, evaluate, and control risk, defined as the organization's risk of accidental financial liability

Role-based access control (RBAC): A control system in which access decisions are based on the roles of individual users as part of an organization

Sale of information: The disclosure of PHI for compensation; HITECH has imposed restrictions on this function

Scalable: The measure of a system to grow relative to various measures of size, speed, number of users, volume of data, and so on

Security: (1) The means to control access and protect information from accidental or intentional disclosure to unauthorized persons and from unauthorized alteration, destruction, or loss; (2) The physical protection of facilities and equipment from theft, damage, or unauthorized access; collectively, the policies, procedures, and safeguards designed to protect the confidentiality of information, maintain the integrity and availability of information systems, and control access to the content of these systems

Self-encrypted hard drives: Hard drives that protect their own data through keys that reside on the drive itself

Shadow records: Duplicate, such as photocopied, records that are maintained separately from the official health record

Single-factor authentication: Use of one of three mechanisms to corroborate the identity of who an individual claims to be; the three mechanisms include (1) what the person knows (such as, password); (2) what the user has (such as, token); and (3) what the user is (such as, biometrics); is less secure than two-factor authentication

Stand-alone authorizations: HIPAA-recognized authorization that does not combine informed consent with authorization to use or disclose PHI

Statute: A piece of legislation written and approved by a state or federal legislature and then signed into law by the state's governor or the president

Subcontractor: An entity that performs work for HIPAA business associates and meets the business associate definition by performing functions or activities on behalf of the business associate involving the use or disclosure of individually identifiable health information; subcontractors are named as business associates in HITECH

System characterization: The first step of risk analysis; it focuses on what the organization possesses by identifying which information assets need protection

Technical safeguards: A set of five standards defined by the HIPAA Security Rule that can be implemented from a technical standpoint using computer software: access controls, audit controls, data integrity, person or entity authentication, and transmission security to protect ePHI

Technology neutral: A characteristic of the HIPAA Security Rule that allows an organization to develop as their technological capabilities allow rather than requiring or prescribing certain technologies

Telemedicine: A telecommunications system that links healthcare organizations and patient from diverse geographic locations and transmits text and images for (medical) consultation and treatment

Text messaging: The electronic exchange of information between mobile electronic devices using a telephone network

Tiered penalties: Civil monetary penalties imposed by HITECH that increase based on levels of intent and neglect; the established tiers are (1) unknowing or did not know; (2) reasonable cause that cannot be identified as willful neglect; and (3) willful neglect, corrected and uncorrected

Transmission security: A HIPAA Security Rule technical safeguard that provides for measures to be taken to protect ePHI against unauthorized access during transmission via an electronic communications network

Treatment: One of three collective functions (the other two being payment and healthcare operations) necessary to successfully conduct business; some of HIPAA's requirements (including patient authorization) are removed or relaxed when an individual's PHI is needed to carry out a treatment function; includes providing, coordinating, or managing healthcare services as well as provider consultations and referrals

Treatment, payment, and healthcare operations (TPO): Term used in the HIPAA Privacy Rule pertaining to broad activities under normal treatment, payment, and operations activities, important because of the rule's many exceptions to the release and disclosure of personal health information. Collectively, these three actions are functions of a covered entity which are necessary for the covered entity to successfully conduct business

Two-factor authentication: Use of two of three mechanisms to corroborate the identity of who an individual claims to be; the three mechanisms include (1) what the person knows (such as, password); (2) what the user has (such as, token); and (3) what the user is (such as, biometrics); is more secure than single-factor authentication

Unconditioned authorizations: A HIPAA-recognized authorization that does not condition the provision of research-related treatment on the presence of an authorization

United States Department of Health and Human Services (HHS): The cabinet-level federal agency that oversees all the health- and human-services-related activities of the federal government and administers federal regulations

Use: The handling of PHI that is internal to a covered entity or business associate including functions such as utilization, examination, and analysis

User-based access control (UBAC): A security mechanism used to grant users of a system access based on identity

Vulnerability: An inherent weakness or absence of a safeguard that could be exploited by a threat

Waived authorization: Results from an IRB or privacy board decision not to require an individual's authorization for use or disclosure of PHI related to a research study

Workforce: Under the HIPAA Privacy Rule, employees, volunteers, trainees, and other persons whether paid or not who work for and are under the direct control of the covered entity

Workstation: A computer designed to accept data from multiple sources in order to assist in managing information for daily activities and to provide a convenient means of entering data as desired by the user at the point of care

Index

ANSI. *See* American National Standards Institute (ANSI)

Anticipated threats, 24, 83, 118, 186

Antivirus software packages, 96

AOA. *See* American Osteopathic Association (AOA)

APA. *See* Administrative Procedure Act (APA)

Applications and data criticality analysis (45 CFR 164.308(a)(7)(ii)(E)), 105

ARRA. *See* American Recovery and Reinvestment Act (ARRA)

Assigned security responsibility (45 CFR 164.308(a)(2)), 100

Association of Rehabilitation Centers, 10

ATLs. *See* Accredited Testing Laboratories (ATLs)

Attorneys General (Section 13410), 158–59

Audit controls (45 CFR 164.312(b)), 90, 93

Audit log, 93, 100, 103, 131

Audit trail, 93, 94, 103, 128, 154

Audits (Section 13411), 159

Authentication, 94, 96

Authorizations
    altered, 72
    compound, 72
    conditioned, 72, 161
    defective, 52
    HIPAA, 50–55
    from patient, 181

Authorization/supervision (45 CFR 164.308(a)(3)(ii)(A)), 100

Automatic fax systems, 187

Automatic log-off (45 CFR 164.312(a)(2)(iii)), 91–92

Availability (45 CFR 164.316(b)(2)(ii)), 109

B

BAA. *See* Business associate agreement (BAA)

BAs. *See* Business associates (BAs)

Baseline identification, 120

Behavioral health notes, 53

Bodies
    accrediting and certifying, 8
    ONC-authorized EHR certification, 12

Breach, 120, 149–50
    report, 151

Breach notification (section 13402), 148–52

"Break the glass," 91, 103

Business associate agreement (BAA), 28–29, 130, 147, 177

Business associate contracts (45 CFR 164.314(a)(2)(i)), 106

Business associate contracts and other arrangements (45 CFR 164.308(b)(1)), 105–6

Business associate contracts or other arrangements (45 CFR 164.314(a)(1)), 106–7

Business associates (BAs), 48, 177
    BAA, 28–29
    breach notification regulations, 150
    covered entities and, 153, 163
    identification, 27
    minimum necessary, 33
    and subcontractors (sections 13401, 13404, 13408), 147–48

Business continuity plan, 126
    and emergency mode of operations, 128–29

C

Cabinet-level federal agency, 143

CAPTA of 1996. *See* Child Abuse Prevention and Treatment Act (CAPTA) of 1996

CARF. *See* Commission on Accreditation of Rehabilitation Facilities (CARF)

CBAC. *See* Context-based access control (CBAC)

CCHIT. *See* Certification Commission for Health Information Technology (CCHIT)

Centers for Medicare and Medicaid Services (CMS), 9–10, 17

Centralized RLS, 133

Certification, 8

Certification Commission for Health Information Technology (CCHIT), 18–19

"Certified EHR Technology," 13, 18

CFR. *See* Code of Federal Regulations (CFR)

Chart tracking functions, 129

Child Abuse Prevention and Treatment Act (CAPTA) of 1996, 6

Cignet Health, 163

Civil monetary penalties, 160

"Clearly and conspicuously," 157

Clinical Laboratory Improvements Amendments (CLIA) of 1988, 66

CMS. *See* Centers for Medicare and Medicaid Services (CMS)

Code of Ethics, violation of, 20

Code of Federal Regulations (45 CFR 160 and 164), 26

ONC. *See* Office of the National Coordinator (ONC)

ONC-AA. *See* Office of the National Coordinator for Health Information Technology-Approved Accreditor (ONC-AA)

ONC-ACBs. *See* Office of the National Coordinator for Health Information Technology-Authorized Certification Bodies (ONC-ACBs)

ONC-ATCBs. *See* Office of the National Coordinator for Health Information Technology-Authorized Testing and Certification Bodies (ONC-ATCBs)

Online breach reporting system, 151

On-site storage, 130

"Opt-in" model, 131

"Opt-out" model, 131

Oral agreement, 161

Organ procurement organizations, 49

Organizational compliance, ensuring, 166

Organizational policy, 20

Organizational requirements (45 CFR 164.314), 83, 106–8

Organized healthcare arrangement, 38

Other arrangements (45 CFR 164.314(a)(2)(ii)), 107

P

Parens patriae power, 158

Password management (45 CFR 164.308 (a)(5)(ii)(D)), 103

Passwords, 94

    secured, tips for, 95

Patient authorization, 55

Patient information, privacy and security of, 128

Patient portal, 133

Patient safety organizations (PSOs), 148

Patients

    financial information, 120

    PHI of, 178

    records, 136

    rights, glance of, 62–65

    sign in for appointments, 184

Payment, 36

Penalty monies, 160

Per HITECH, 153, 157

Person authentication (45 CFR 164.312(d)), 94–96

Personal health record (PHR), 133

    vendors section 13407, 156

Personal health record portals, 133

Personal health record vendors, 148

Personal representative of HIPAA, 33

Personnel records, health information in, 38

PHI. *See* Protected health information (PHI)

PHR. *See* Personal health record (PHR)

Physical safeguards (45 CFR 164.310), 83, 84

    device and media controls (45 CFR 164.310(d)(1)), 87–89

    facility access controls (45 CFR 164.310 (a)(1)), 84–86

    workstation security (45 CFR 164.310 (c)), 87

    workstation use (45 CFR 164.310 (b)), 86–87

Physical security, 128

PKI. *See* Public key infrastructure (PKI)

Policies

    organization's internal, 20

    and procedures, 33, 69, 74–75, 86–88, 101–2

Policies and procedures (45 CFR 164.316 (a)), 108

Portable devices, 151

PPOs. *See* Preferred provide organizations (PPOs)

Preemption, 5–6, 61

Preferred provide organizations (PPOs), 10

Privacy

    in HIPAA, 24–26

    measures for HIEs, 132

    program, oversight of, 165

    screens, 185–86

    in semiprivate rooms, 184–85

Privacy Act of 1974, 3–4

Privacy board, 72

Privacy officer, 75

    compliance, 165–66

    daily operations, 166

    privacy expertise, 166–67

    responsibilities, 165

    skills and requirements, 167

Privacy Rule, 161

    HIPAA, 4–7

Private entities, 131

Private key infrastructure, 92, 97

Professional ethical standards, 20

Professional integrity, 167

Promulgation, 143

Proposed rules, 142, 143, 153, 160–61

Protected health information (PHI), 28–30, 33, 147, 148

Protected health information
    (PHI) *(continued)*
    access to own, 61, 66
    amendment to, 67–68
    breach notification, 150–51
    confidential communications of, 69–70
    covered entity and, 57
    of decedents, 161
    electronic, 153
    for marketing, 70
    messaging service software, 186
    NPP, 46–50
    of patients, 178
    privacy of, 47
    public interest and benefit circumstances,
        57–60
    use and disclosure, authorization
        requirements for, 56
    workforce training in, 75
Protection from malicious software (45 CFR
    164.308(a)(5)(ii)(B)), 102–3
Protection of human subjects (45 CFR Part
    46(a)), 71
Provider-to-patient communication, 134
Provider-to-provider communication,
    133, 134
PSOs. *See* Patient safety organizations
    (PSOs)
Psychotherapy notes, 53, 176
Public accounting firm, 159
Public comments, 144
Public entities, 131
Public health, 49
    activities, 7, 58
    disclosure, 161
    reporting, 6–7
Public Health Service Act, 25
Public key infrastructure (PKI), 92
Punitive approach, 163

Q
Qualitative approach, 124, 125
Quantitative approach, 124, 125

R
RBAC. *See* Role-based access control
    (RBAC)
Record locator service (RLS), 133
Red flags, 121
Red Flags Rule, 121
Regional health information organizations
    (RHIOs), 133

Regulations, 143
Religious affiliation, 182
Renewal of ONC-ACB designation, 19
Request, PHI, 36
Required specification, 84
Research Authorization Requirements, 161
Research, HIPAA, 71–74
    use/disclose, PHI for, 59
Residual risks, 125
Response and reporting (45 CFR 164.308
    (a)(6)(ii)), 103–4
Restricted health information, requirements
    for authorization to, 52
Restriction, deidentification, 60
Restriction requests, 69
    Section 13405, 152–53
Results documentation, 124–25
Retaliation, 76
Retraining sessions, routine, 102
Retranscribing documents, 131
RHIOs. *See* Regional health information
    organizations (RHIOs)
Risk analysis
    control recommendations, 124
    impact analysis, 123–24
    likelihood determination, 123
    and management, 117
    reports, documenting, 124
    results documentation, 124–25
    risk determination, 124
    system characterization, 117–18
    threats, identifying, 118–21
    vulnerabilities, identifying, 121–22
Risk analysis (45 CFR 164.308(a)(1)(ii)
    (A)), 99
Risk assessment, breach notification, 150
Risk determination, 124
Risk management (45 CFR 164.308(a)(1)(ii)
    (B)), 99, 104
Risk profiles, 124–25
RLS. *See* Record locator service (RLS)
Robust system, 110
Role-based access control (RBAC), 86, 100
Routine retraining sessions, 102
Rulemaking, types of, 143

S
Sale of information (section 13405), 158
Sanction policy (45 CFR 164.308(a)(1)(ii)
    (C)), 99
Sanctions, 75
Scalable, 83